Defeating Pain

The War Against a Silent Epidemic

Defeating Pain

The War Against a Silent Epidemic

Dr. Patrick D. Wall
and
Mervyn Jones

Plenum Press • New York and London

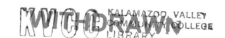

Library of Congress Cataloging-in-Publication Data

Wall, Patrick D.
    Defeating pain : the war against a silent epidemic / Patrick D.
Wall and Mervyn Jones.
        p.   cm.
    Includes bibliographical references and index.
    ISBN 0-306-43964-6
    1. Pain.   I. Jones, Mervyn.   II. Title.
    [DNLM: 1. Pain--etiology. 2. Pain--therapy.   WL 704 W187d]
RB127.W35 1991
616'.0472--dc20
DNLM/DLC
for Library of Congress   91-21359
                                                               CIP

ISBN 0-306-43964-6

© 1991 Patrick D. Wall and Mervyn Jones
Plenum Press is a division of Plenum Publishing Corporation
233 Spring Street, New York, N.Y. 10013

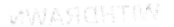

Dedicated to
Those who are in pain and to those who help them

and to Robert Wald, who had the idea of an
International Pain Foundation.

Contents

Introduction 1
Chapter 1   The Silent Epidemic 7
Chapter 2   The Causes of Pain 31
Chapter 3   Childbirth: Pain without Illness 69
Chapter 4   Paradoxes of Pain 91
Chapter 5   Mechanisms of Pain 109
Chapter 6   The Unanswered Cry 141
Chapter 7   Pain Behavior 153
Chapter 8   Treatment of Pain with Medicine 167
Chapter 9   Therapy by Surgery, Restoration, or
             Stimulation 191
Chapter 10   Belief-and-Attitude Therapies 215
Chapter 11   Fighting Against Pain 235
Chapter 12   Lessons and Prospects 253
References 271
Further Reading 275
Index 277

Introduction

To state the obvious, pain is an unpleasant subject. Large numbers of people in every country on earth have to endure frequent, even incessant pain; still larger numbers are obligatory spectators of the pain endured by those they love. These people may turn with interest to a book about pain, which should bring a sympathetic consideration of the problems it poses. We trust that they will not be disappointed, for we have kept them very much in mind while writing this book. But they may also feel, understandably, that living with pain is bad enough without also reading thousands of words about it. Perhaps a book on this unpleasant subject will itself be merely unpleasant and depressing.

We wish to say at the outset, therefore, that we have written in a spirit of well-grounded optimism. The world possesses far greater resources for the alleviation, and in some circumstances the elimination, of pain than at any time in the past. We shall describe in detail what these resources are and how they have evolved. It is reasonable to expect, moreover, that resources for fighting pain will be extended and strengthened in the future. If our book has a message, it is a message of hope.

The causes of this gratifying situation are both technical and intellectual. Technically, medical professionals are now equipped to combat pain with increasingly delicate surgical procedures, with a greatly enlarged pharmacological repertoire, and by methods such as electrical stimulation, which have been developed recently and are still being improved. These will be discussed in chapters devoted to the treatment of pain. The intellectual progress—it would not be too much to call it an intellectual revolution—is more complex, but perhaps even more remarkable and significant.

Progress in science does not come about by chance, or entirely thanks to the appearance of an individual genius. It requires the development, or perhaps the creation, of adequate research institutions and university departments. It also requires a career choice by a sufficient number of people exceptionally endowed with intelligence and creative originality. At a certain point in history, one branch of science or another is seen to be "exciting" and benefits by being thus seen. In the mid-nineteenth century it was geology; later, physics and mathematics held pride of place. In our own age, the life sciences—biology, biochemistry, genetics—are generally conceded to be the exciting sphere and have consequently made the swiftest progress.

It also happens that a branch of knowledge that was hardly taken seriously can gain respect, and be virtually transformed, in a fairly short space of time. The casual observation of the habits of "primitive peoples" by explorers was thus transformed into the science of anthropology. Random treasure hunting in Greece and Italy was the foundation of archaeology. The precursors of modern psychiatry were doctors, known as alienists, who had the job of keeping the insane in confinement and in moderately decent conditions, without any attempt at treatment. Similarly, there was a time—not much more than 50 years ago—when a doctor who concerned himself primarily with the treatment of pain would have been regarded as either very humble in his aspirations or eccentric to the point of absurdity.

The reasoning was that, since pain was an inevitable accompaniment of certain recognized conditions (cancer, angina pectoris, arthritis), relief of pain was impossible, or possible only to a very limited extent. Therefore, it was merely the business of a junior nurse, if the patient was in a hospital, or a member of the family in other situations. Training was scarcely necessary, nor was an understanding of the pain process within the human body. The doctor had more important things to think about. In scientific terms, pain was irrelevant.

As we shall see when we take a closer look at the medical scene, this traditional attitude is not altogether extinct. The diffusion of knowledge about the problems of pain and the emphasis placed on them in medical education fall decidedly short of desirable levels. There has, nevertheless, been a considerable change. Very few doctors under the age of 40 would now dismiss the subject of pain in the fashion just described. A doctor who announces that pain is his main interest can hope to be viewed with respect by his compeers. He or she can look forward to working in a pain clinic (the proliferation of these clinics in the last 20 years is a notable sign of the changed atmosphere) or with a research team, and thus to an advancement in status, which doctors value at least as much as anyone else. In short, pain is being taken seriously. The rise in the esteem of pain studies has led, as one would expect, to an increase in the fruitfulness of these studies.

This change of attitude in the medical profession has proceeded alongside a similar change among the population at large, at least in developed countries where scientific progress is feasible. As in other contexts, the disentangling of cause and effect is an intricate matter. However, resignation to the inevitability of pain is no longer the prevailing mood, whether of the sufferers themselves, of their families and friends, or of thinking people in general. On the contrary, the predominant view is that pain is a problem to be tackled, both on a social scale and in each individual case. The more widely and the more strongly this view is held, the more we can look forward to its being tackled effectively.

Although we are now in the realm of speculation, we can suggest several reasons for the change. One of these is the weakening of the belief that pain is ordained by a power above and beyond our comprehension and is "in the nature of things." Traditionally, this belief has been associated with the Christian religion. Yet it is precisely in Christian (or nominally Christian) countries that scientific discovery has given us greater control over our environment and a greater ability to combat ancient scourges. In the twentieth century, inherited doctrines about the necessity of pain and the virtues of resignation have been largely abandoned by modern-minded clerics and believers. It may well be God's will, they would say, that doctors should achieve a growing capacity to deal with pain. Thus, the simplistic beliefs of the past are inevitably losing their hold.

Meanwhile, the problem of avoidable suffering has become a central concern for all thinking people. The dominant images of suffering on a mass scale, evoked by Auschwitz and Hiroshima, have left an ineradicable mark on our consciousness. There is no direct link between the final terrifying moments in the gas chambers and the agony of a terminal cancer patient waiting for an overdue morphine injection, but the common theme is our revulsion against helpless suffering. We seem to have accepted an obligation to atone for remembered acts of cruelty and callousness by resolving to prevent any suffering of which we are aware.

As time passes and softens the outlines of the past, we are tempted to look back nostalgically to the safe, civilized world of the era that ended in 1914. Wars were brief, localized, and quite romantic, while horrors such as the extermination of entire peoples were undreamed of. But we forget the callousness toward individual suffering that was hidden beneath this smooth surface. As already mentioned, the care of the mentally ill was merely custodial and sometimes ruthlessly brutal. In fact, there is considerable evidence for the optimistic view that in our lifetime, the world has become progressively more humane. Resources (not enough, to be sure, but better than nothing) are devoted to children who are spastic, brain-damaged, or affected by Down's syndrome; not so long ago these children were dismissed as hopelessly "defective." Old people who used to be pitied, or indeed ridiculed, as "gaga" are now recognized as having Alzheimer's disease. Facilities for the disabled are a social obligation; in the past, these people scarcely ventured out of doors. In all these cases, greater knowledge and understanding have gone together with greater compassion. Because we have achieved an insight into, for instance, the minds of the autistic, we are able to do something for them—but it is equally true to say that, because we care, we have sought the knowledge. In the complexity of human life, there are still mysteries and unsolved problems, but experience encourages us to believe that there are no problems which cannot be solved.

This is the climate that has produced the new attitude toward pain. We are no longer content to accept the bleak, dismissive dictum that, while some people are blind and some are deaf, some are doomed to endless pain. That outlook both generated and confirmed a refusal to analyze and investigate pain—to *think* about pain. As soon as scientifically trained minds were directed toward purposeful thinking, the results were startling in their novelty and impressive in their scope.

We shall see in the course of this book that most of the obvious, common-sense beliefs about pain, taken for granted over the centuries, have been discredited by investigation. It was "obvious" that, just as some nerves transmit sensations of heat or cold, other nerves transmit pain—obvious, but untrue. It was "obvious" that pain was proportionate to physical injury, so that a major injury caused grave pain while a minor injury caused slight pain—again, obvious, but untrue. The study of pain reminds us that the function of science is to subject accepted belief to scrutiny. It was once "obvious," let us remember, that malaria was caused by bad air.

The fundamental reason why knowledge about pain was so limited, and indeed so faulty and inaccurate, was that it was not regarded as a medical problem at all, but merely a phenomenon sometimes associated with medical problems. The starting point of present-day research is to confront pain as a problem in its own right. Given this approach, it is not really surprising that research has produced a vastly increased understanding of the nature, cause, and possible treatment of pain. Not surprising, perhaps—but highly gratifying.

To place this new understanding and knowledge in the hands of interested readers is the aim of this book.

1

The Silent Epidemic

As we travel the highways or ride the city buses, we often see posters and advertisements pleading for contributions to research into cancer, heart disease, muscular dystrophy, and other threats to health. Other posters warn of the dangers of AIDS, the newest scourge; and the traditional appeals to help the blind and the deaf are still prominent. These are all good causes that unquestionably merit our support. Yet, the most widespread and intractable of all health problems is mentioned in none of the posters. It is pain.

In the United States and in other nations with a comparable standard of living, we can estimate that one adult in every six is suffering from pain at any given moment. Twenty million Americans are in pain from arthritis; 30 million, seven million of whom are wholly or partially disabled, have endured spells of persistent back pain at some time in their lives; and millions more are in pain from cancer, angina pectoris, and other causes. No single sickness comes anywhere near equaling pain in the sheer scale of incidence.

PAIN AS AN EPIDEMIC

To consider and study pain as an epidemic can bring answers to many questions and cast doubt on many fallacies. For example, some people accept the high incidence of pain in the United States without surprise because they have a simple explanation: America is the epitome of a high-stress culture, characterized by unhealthy lifestyles and an unhealthy environment.

In 1985 a useful survey of the incidence of pain in the United States was carried out, examining a sample of the entire population over the age of 18 (65). The reason for this survey was that a pharmaceutical company, Bristol-Myers, was about to introduce a new analgesic (that is, a drug for pain alleviation), Nuprin, and thus wished to understand the extent of the problem. The results confirmed the high incidence of pain complaints. Fifteen percent of the sample, 26 million people, had suffered backache for over 31 days in the previous year. Some 30% of these people rated their backaches as severe or crippling. Can we explain away these numbers by saying that the sufferers are overweight, inactive, overdrinking, oversmoking slobs? No; large numbers among them are model citizens. Of the sample, 18% jogged, 34% exercised regularly, 70% did not smoke, and 78% were very moderate drinkers (less than six drinks a week).

Should we, then, point the finger at stress rather than at unhealthy living? Richard Sternbach, a pioneer in the study of the psychology of pain at the Scripps Clinic in La Jolla, California, made a survey on this question in 1986 (61, 62). People suffering from various types of pain were asked what they considered to be the main cause of the pain. The answers were:

Headaches	39% named stress as main cause
Menstrual pain	35%
Stomach pain	7%
Backaches	4%

Sternbach then surveyed a sample of the general population, asking them whether they rated the stress in their lives as high or low, and what pain (if any) they had suffered from for more than 31 days in the previous year. The findings were:

	Low stress	High stress
Headaches	7%	25%
Backaches	12%	25%
Muscle pains	7%	13%
Joint pains	13%	27%
Stomach pains	4%	14%
Menstrual pain (over 11 days)	14%	32%
Dental pain	2%	7%

These are the first clear figures on the relation of stress to pain in large numbers of people. To confirm the results, a special investigation was made of 165 people under heavy stress, such as New York advertising executives and stock exchange floor traders. The greater the stress, it was found, the greater was the liability to pain.

Should we now conclude that stress is the cause of pain? Absolutely not! If we look again at the people who were under low stress, we see that backache affected a far from negligible 12%. Furthermore, even among the high-stress group, Stern-bach insists that a correlation does not prove a cause. Pain itself is obviously a cause of stress, so the correlation can work either way. We have introduced these details here in order to emphasize a major theme of this book: the psychological factor is necessarily a significant component of pain, but only on rare and special occasions is it the only component. We shall be continually exploring the relative roles of injury, damage, or disease and of attitudes, thinking, and brain processes.

There will be those—particularly American readers, perhaps—who will not be impressed by American statistics because they will say that low stress levels in the United States are still pretty awful. But although international comparisons are difficult because of varying diagnostic criteria, figures from other countries are remarkably similar.

Migraine is particularly interesting because many people attribute it to stress when they observe it in others. Migraine sufferers often have a quite different attitude. The condition has been surveyed in a large variety of countries and communities (11). Among 4000 7-year-old children in Finland, 3.2% had migraine, and there was no difference in the rate between boys and girls. By the time this group reached the age of 14, migraine affected 14.8% of the girls and 6.4% of the boys. In a survey of 2000 Danish people aged 40, 18% of the women, but only 8% of the men, suffered from migraine. Evidently age and sex play an important role.

The recognition of pain in children has been a grossly neglected subject, only now receiving serious attention (36, 37). A major problem is the child's limited means of expression. An awful mistake made by doctors and nurses is to confuse frozen terror and learned helplessness with quiet acceptance.

Many people try to believe that somewhere in the world there is a perfect nirvana free from hassles and stress. Sad to say, no such pain-free zone has ever been discovered. Among Nigerian university students, presumably under heavy stress as they prepared for exams, 3% of men and 6% of women were found to suffer from migraine. But when a survey using the same diagnostic criteria was made of people of all ages in the presumably tranquil scene of rural Nigeria, the figures actually rose to 5% of men and 9% of women. Castaways on desert islands have not been surveyed, but it is a fair bet that if they had anyone to complain to, they would.

Statistics from medical sources are bound to underestimate the amount of pain. Undoubtedly, many people decide to "grin and bear it" when afflicted by intermittent pain, or else to rely on simple pain relievers, such as aspirin, bought at the drugstore. In one survey, 75% of Americans reported that they had had headaches on at least one day in the preceding year, while 12% had had headaches—severe in many cases—on 31 or more days (65). Some people in quite severe pain have given up seeking relief and come to the conclusion that no doctor can do anything for them. Some put their faith in unorthodox health techniques and unqualified practitioners, or simply in prayer. Some, in a country that lacks a free and universal health service, cannot seek treatment that would be beyond their means. According to the Nuprin survey, 18% of people who described their pain as severe or unbearable had never sought professional help.

A recent survey investigated all the 128 medical students, with an average age of 21 years, attending a London medical school. Various types of pain were revealed, roughly to the same extent as among other people. These young men and women had completely free access to excellent medical care and were in personal contact with medical staff members. Despite this, many had never consulted a physician, although they suffered from pain that interrupted their work. The explanations varied from passive acceptance to fear of being labeled weak, hysterical, or hypochondriac. They represented the type of person who accepts pain as an inevitable fact of life, to be borne stoically and privately. This illustrates another major theme of this book: the need to differentiate between public display and private suffering. The relation between the two varies widely depending on the particular situation, on personality, and on culture. When the amount of public display seems inappropriate to the amount of disease or damage, we have to consider the pain complaint with a completely open mind. We must not leap to the conclusion that pain complaints are nothing but a public show.

Pain also represents an enormous economic cost to a developed society. In the United States, this cost has been reckoned—as a total of medical expenses, lost income, lost productivity, and compensation payments—at an annual $50 billion. This figure too, because of the extent of unreported pain, is sure to understate the reality. It is impossible to know how many people at work, when in pain, perform at less than normal capacity, lose concentration, snatch rest periods, make hasty or ill-considered decisions, forget important pieces of information, or cause accidents through inattention and clumsiness. In this book, we are less concerned with global economic losses than with the avoidable suffering of living, individual human beings. But the undermining of the sense of achievement, reflected in the satisfaction of doing things well and reliably, is itself a part of the distress that goes with being in pain.

The problem of pain would be less formidable, though still extremely serious, if we could claim that its dimensions are being reduced. In developed nations, the diseases regarded as major threats to health are being more or less successfully conquered by a combination of medical progress, higher living standards, and an improved environment. Some—such as tuberculosis, diphtheria, and polio—are now rarities. But pain is not diminishing either in its incidence, in its duration, or in the scale of the suffering it causes. Indeed, it is on the increase. More people are in pain now than ever before in history.

A major cause of this trend is the aging of the population. In developed nations, life expectancy has risen from about 50 at the beginning of this century to over 70 at the present time. People classed as elderly or old (wherever one chooses to draw the line) therefore constitute a much larger segment of the population than ever before. Thanks to improved medical standards, many are in good health, but many are not. They tend to be affected by conditions such as osteoarthritis, which pose no danger to life but cause persistent pain. Typically, osteoarthritis makes its appearance at some time after the age of 50 and steadily becomes more painful and incapacitating. A sufferer who lives beyond the age of 80 may thus have endured 30 years of pain. We could point out to these people that they would probably be dead if they had lived in the nineteenth century, but that is unlikely to bring much comfort.

Modern medicine has succeeded in extending life well beyond the point at which, in the past, death would have appeared inevitable and natural. People with poorly functioning hearts are kept going by pacemakers. People with diseased kidneys spend 2 days a week on dialysis or receive a transplant. Unfortunately, extending life is not the same thing as restoring normal health. The price of survival is recurrent strain, which expresses itself through spells of pain.

A century ago, someone who developed cancer could be expected to die within a short time. Fifty years ago, there were two possible prospects: one was death, and the other was successful elimination of the cancer, generally by surgery or radiotherapy. Today there is a third possibility: the cancer is "fought," as doctors say, and is held in check by various techniques of treatment, so that the patient survives for 8 to 10 years, until the cancer eventually wins the battle.

Fortunately—and contrary to widespread fears—cancer is not always painful. Some 30% of patients with advanced cancers do not suffer from pain (1). Of those who do, over 90% obtain adequate control over the pain, thanks to the remarkable advances in care and medication made in recent years. The subject of pain in cancer is one that we shall discuss later in detail. The point to be made in the present context is that the greater longevity of cancer patients is related to the general problem of the rising incidence of pain.

Another large and growing category of people in pain consists of those who have survived serious injuries. We are understandably shocked when we think of the numbers of people who, a century ago, lost their lives as a result of fires, industrial accidents, train crashes, or mining disasters. Before the age of the car, the telephone, and the radio, it took much longer for a doctor on horseback to reach the scene of an accident, or for an injured man to be taken to the hospital. Medical and surgical techniques were rudimentary by our standards. When there were no blood transfusions, people bled to death. When there were no skin grafts, people died from the effects of extensive burns. By contrast, modern medicine and intensive care can often preserve life in the most difficult conditions.

In warfare, by far the greatest killers were not the bullets but the bacteria. Of those casualties still alive when they reached forward hospitals in World War I, well over 50% subsequently died, almost entirely of uncontrollable infection. By the time of the Vietnam War, this number had fallen to 5% despite the fact that rapid evacuation now brought much more serious surviving casualties to hospitals.

In all this, there is cause for satisfaction with the progress achieved. What we sometimes forget, however, is that the damaged and repaired body may live in pain long after the rescue operation. It must also be borne in mind that, unlike the victims of arthritis or cancer, people injured in accidents are predominantly young. The paraplegic in a wheelchair may have been a mountain climber or a steeplechase rider. He may be in pain for most of his waking hours from the age of 20 to the age of 80.

The pain that follows an amputation is particularly distressing. In a survey of 29,000 American amputees who were still alive in the 1980s, 7% were found to be in severe pain. Six months after the Yom Kippur War of 1973, an investigation was made of the 186 Israeli soldiers who had suffered amputations (13). They had survived their massive injuries thanks to efficient first aid in battlefield areas, rapid evacuation, and excellent hospital care—but their pain had also survived and resisted treatment. Ten percent were in pain shortly after the amputation—and the same 10% were in pain when reexamined between 5 and 8 years later.

Thus, by a cruel irony, pain is a by-product of the successes of medicine. The professional ethos absorbed by every medical student teaches that a doctor's supreme duty is to save or prolong life, even when the chances of recovery are very slender or indeed nonexistent. A doctor would feel culpable if he refrained from applying a treatment because he could foresee the aftermath of pain. In any case, the surgeon who amputates the leg or performs the skin grafts does not bear the responsibility for alleviating the pain that lingers for years after the patient has left the hospital.

In the most famous New York cancer hospital, some 20% of the patients' pains were listed as iatrogenic—that is, caused by the medical or surgical treatment the patients received (22). Leaving aside those that resulted from medical errors (doctors are human and fallible), the treatment causing the pain was the outcome of a difficult decision, embodying a calculated balance of advantage and danger. Naturally, this topic is about as popular with doctors as the casualty rate is with generals.

To put the established medical ethos into reverse would be both wrong and impossible. The proper response to this enormous incidence of pain is to recognize it for what it is: the greatest health problem of our age. This means that the effort to relieve the suffering caused by pain—through the work of doctors and other health professionals in individual cases, and also through research into the fundamentals of the problems—should receive the priority, and be supported by the resources, that were given in the past to the major disease problems. Fortunately, a considerable shift of emphasis in this direction has taken place in the last 20 years.

WHY DOES SOCIETY IGNORE PAIN?

This question is so important that we shall be devoting a chapter to exploring it. Here, we can summarize the advances of recent years.

Helen Neal is prominent among those who have drawn public attention to the problem. In a book that at first received little publicity, she coined the phrase "the silent epidemic of pain" (51). The history of her interest in the subject is illuminating. In 1964 her brother began to suffer pain, caused partly by tongue cancer and partly by the treatment he had received. She was working at the National Institutes of Health (NIH) in Bethesda, Maryland, which is by far the largest research center for medical problems anywhere in the world. Furthermore, it organizes the financing of the bulk of biomedical research in the universities and hospitals of the United States and has special programs in many other countries. It is in fact a group of institutes, each dedicated to special health and disease areas. These subdivisions reflect the accepted consensus of society as expressed by pressure groups of doctors, charities, politicians, and citizens. There are institutes for heart disease, cancer, stroke, blindness, alcoholism, and so on. But there is no institute for pain. Even today, the NIH finances only two relatively small programs dedicated to the conquest of pain.

Helen Neal searched the vast organization for someone who could help her brother and found no one. Even worse, there was little interest in her questions. Outside the NIH, she did discover that developments were in slow progress. She found a very sympathetic ear in Professor John Bonica of Seattle, who had been battling for years to persuade physicians and surgeons to pay attention to pain and to try to mobilize efforts to control pain. In 1953 he had written a pioneering book that had slowly penetrated into the practice of doctors, particularly his fellow anesthesiologists (7).

Today, the historical neglect of the problem is being replaced by clearly visible movement. When those who suffer began to rise in revolt, the medical profession showed signs of accepting responsibility and basic scientists reexamined the problem. In the early 1970s, physicians such as Bonica joined with scientists to form the International Association for the Study of Pain. It now has a membership of 4000, half in North America and about 30% in Western Europe. But this welcome development is a luxury limited to developed nations; there are only 34 members in the Arab nations, 30 in India, two in Pakistan, and none in the whole of Central Africa or Central America.

A monthly professional journal, *Pain*, was founded in 1975 and now has 5000 hospital, university, and individual subscribers. There are growing numbers of journals and of national professional societies. But charity organizations dedicated to encouraging information, education, training, and research on the subject of pain remain astonishingly rare. In the United

States, a single fund, the International Pain Foundation, is young and struggling. In Britain, a single charity concentrates on supporting one research group. We know of none in the rest of Europe.

If we wish to understand why so many doctors over several generations have regarded pain as unimportant and uninteresting, we have to look first at the aims and priorities of modern medicine. These were firmly established in the early nineteenth century and accepted by physicians and patients alike. The aim of medicine today is fundamental diagnosis of the cause of disease and treatment to eliminate that cause. In the eighteenth century, there were no such precise pretensions. For example, in 1763 the Reverend Edmund Stone communicated what turned out to be a key paper to the Royal Society. It announced the discovery of the effect of willow bark, from which later work derived aspirin and a large family of analgesics. However, he writes that it is "very efficacious in curing anguish and intermitting disorders." By "curing," he meant relief of the symptoms, fever and pain. One hundred years later, with Pasteur and Virchow and the other giants in full cry, "curing" meant elimination of cause, not manipulation of signs and symptoms. Beyond argument, this shift of emphasis was immensely constructive.

Let us take the example of malaria, still one of the world's major debilitators and killers. In Napoleonic times, the cause of malaria was seen as exposure to the miasma of damp swamp night air. This was correct in the vaguest sort of way. The cure at that time was quinine. That was also correct in an astonishingly serendipitous way. South American Indians had discovered, in the extraordinary way of folk cultures to link cause and effect, that the bark of the cinchona tree helped some people with severe fevers. It turned out that quinine poisoned the *Plasmodium* parasite that causes malaria slightly more effectively than it poisoned the people who harbor the parasite. Suppose that nineteenth- and twentieth-century physicians and scientists had decided that the real problem with people with malaria lay in signs and symptoms, i.e., sweating, fever, rigors, headaches, and so on. Suppose that malaria research had concentrated on the control of such signs and symptoms. We would know nothing of the fact that mosquitoes are the essence of the night air or that they transmit a protozoon. We would know nothing of the parasite, or of quinine, or of the compounds that can better attack the parasite. Malaria remains a serious problem, but the diagnosis is now exact, cures are frequent, prevention is conceivable, and final victory is more a social–political problem than a technical one.

This story can be repeated for many diseases. Such are the genuine triumphs of the shift to science. With the change of attitude, a new hierarchy was established in the medical profession. At the top of the heap were the new action men among the physicians and surgeons. If cancer is diagnosed, the patient and his doctor seek first a surgeon to cut it out and eliminate it. If the cancer is too widespread for surgical excision, the oncologist moves in with the magic bullets of radiation or chemicals that kill dividing cells.

Other specialties were rather less prestigious. Neurologists developed intellectually impressive ways of diagnosing precisely what was wrong with the brain, but were not concerned with cures. Psychiatrists contributed methods of interpretation which, by their nature, were less precise. Then came the physiotherapists, nurses, and social workers, who attempted neither diagnosis nor cure—they simply helped people.

Patients, meanwhile, became more sophisticated in their attitudes. They rejected treatments such as analgesics, which not only failed to cure, but could actually submerge useful signs and symptoms. The phrase "symptomatic medicine" became synonymous with "bad medicine." It was regarded as a concentration on signposts diverting doctors and patients from their logical progress along a road to a clear end. Coupled with the age of reason in medicine was a suspicion of pragmatic medicine. If something worked but lacked an evident rationale, it was condemned. Hence a growing suspicion of herbs that had not been analyzed, of soothsayers, necromancers, and manipulators, and of everything that has now come to be called alternative medicine. Yet this type of traditional medicine has withstood both the test of time and the assaults of modern orthodox medicine.

The historical progress from classical symptomatic medicine to modern diagnose-and-cure medicine has not been without counteractions. One of these is homeopathy, originally known as Hahnemannism because the pioneer of the technique was the German physician Samuel Hahnemann (1755–1843), a respected figure after whom the Philadelphia medical school is named. Homeopathy is now associated with the use of unusual compounds in greatly diluted concentrations. However, Hahnemann's aim was to return to treating the details of what made the patient suffer, paying attention to the signs and symptoms that were being neglected by the new doctors. His approach was to seek compounds which, in high concentration, actually produced the signs and symptoms. The theory, which is correct in some cases, is that a compound that produces a symptom in high concentrations produces the opposite in low concentrations. This explains the origin of the word "homeopathy," which means treatment with the same (*homeo*) compound that produces the disease (*pathy*).

These counteractions have been growing and persisting. It is becoming accepted that, while awaiting the definitive solution of diagnosis and cure, it is not contradictory to seek and even demand symptom control. Many groups are concerned with paraplegic patients with spinal cord damage. For some, the only aim is cure, which will require a solution of the unsolved problem of how to get nerve fibers in the spinal cord to grow and to seek the correct target, as they did in the embryo. Others, however, try to relieve particularly distressing conditions: pain, faulty bladder function, muscle contraction, and so on. Astonishingly bitter battles rage in which each side accuses the other of gullibility and of wasting resources. This is sad, for the two sides are complementary rather than antagonistic, although it is quite true that resources are inadequate.

People in pain and those who care for them are also rising up in revolt against their enforced passive waiting until a cure appears. One reaction is to search the classical folk remedies abandoned by modern medicine. Another reaction is to demand better day-to-day care of the patient, which is another way of describing control of symptoms, principally pain. Until fairly recently, such day-to-day care was left as it had stood in the eighteenth century and took no part in the extraordinary advances in thinking and knowledge since that time. In our time, symptomatic treatment has progressed not only by reviving the old values of tender loving care and humanity, but also by mobilizing the skills of thought, analysis, and synthesis, which have improved diagnosis and cure.

In our rational society, we like to believe that there are no sacred cows or taboos. Taboos have an aura of magic, and we all know that magic does not belong in the modern world. Hence, death itself is no longer to be feared so much as the manner of dying. We perceive, predict, and fear that we must inevitably face a period of helpless agony and anguish before death itself, which is seen as a welcome relief. The common phrase in obituaries "died peacefully" is meant as a reassurance, but enhances unspoken fear in those who observe that the phrase is sometimes missing. The persistent dark fear is expressed by relatives of battle casualties who seek the details of death. Every doctor has experienced the hushed awe of the relative whose first question is not "Why did he die?" but "How did he die?" The subject of pain has within it a chilling air of impending horror. For many, it is so deep, inexplicable, and overwhelming, that any mention of the topic is taboo. It seems best to put pain out of mind, not to turn attention to it.

Perhaps, therefore, the neglect of pain—by the medical profession and by society at large—is less surprising than it appears at first glance. It is, nevertheless, based on spurious logic and on ignorance or misunderstanding of important facts. We wrote this book to dispel that ignorance and to contribute toward the recognition and hence the overcoming of pain.

Before we can begin to defeat pain, however, we must understand it. Just as scientists once asked, "What is heart failure?" or "What is cancer?" we need to ask, "What is pain?"

WHAT IS PAIN?

At first glance, the question may seem simple or even pointless. Surely, we all know what pain is. "I am in pain" is a message that can be conveyed by a groan or a shriek, without the need for a common language, and indeed by a baby too young to have acquired language. Yet if we attempt, as an intellectual exercise, to explain what pain means—as though speaking to some fortunate person who has never met with it— we are likely to find the task surprisingly difficult. Edmund Burke, certainly a distinguished thinker, confessed himself beaten and wrote, "Pain and pleasure are simple ideas incapable of definition." We can say, "Pain is a very unpleasant feeling" or "Pleasure is a very enjoyable feeling," but such statements are really tautologies.

One incontestable fact gives us a useful starting point: there is no pain without the consciousness of pain. Undergoing an operation might be horribly painful if you were conscious, but is painless once you are anesthetized. This fact establishes a basic distinction between disease and pain. After making an investigation and examining X-rays, a doctor may tell a patient, "You have cancer." Assuming the evidence to be adequate, this statement is true and will remain true even if the patient finds it incredible and denies it. But if the doctor were to say, "You are in pain," the patient could quite reasonably reply, "No, I'm not." In practice, the doctor knows that the patient is in pain only when the latter says so or demonstrates it by some gesture or reaction. The conclusion is that while a disease can be objectively observed, pain is subjectively experienced.

Now we can ask, "What is the nature of this experience?" We commonly say, "I feel a pain in my eyes" (or my stomach, or my left ear) and it would seem to follow that the experience is purely physical. However, "feel" is a verb that has a broad range of uses. We say, "I feel hot" or "I feel cold"; we also say, "I feel happy" or "I feel sad." This suggests that feeling pain may be a somewhat complex experience.

We have an immensely rich language and, needless to say, have a rich vocabulary related to the subject of pain. On the most mundane level, television commercials use the phrase "minor aches and pains." If the television allows you time to think, you might ask, "What is the difference between an ache and a pain?" It would be distracting and cheating to look the words up in a dictionary. Most people would probably say that they are similar but a pain is worse than an ache. This question of exactly how people use words to describe their pains became a particular interest of Ronald Melzack, now Professor of Psychology at McGill University in Montreal. He was a postdoctoral fellow in the 1950s and fortuitously (and fortunately for us) came under the influence of W. K. Livingston in Portland, Oregon. Livingston, a professor of neurosurgery in the neighboring state of Washington, slightly older than Bonica, had been in charge of the human wreckage shipped back from the Pacific battlegrounds during World War II with nerve injuries. In 1943 he had written a book (32) that reexamined the very problems Weir Mitchell had explored in 1872 after seeing other young Americans wounded in the Civil War. Livingston maintained his interest in pain problems, and following the Hippocratic tradition of good medicine, taught Melzack to look at patients and to listen to what they say. This tradition is often forgotten by a new breed of high-tech doctors and patients who want a computer printout of machine measures. For 15 years, Melzack patiently recorded the words used by patients in pain (40).

He compiled a collection of words that he divided into four categories: (1) sensory—words used to describe the kind of pain that was felt; (2) affective—words used to convey the nature of the experience; (3) evaluative—words used to rate the pain according to its severity. Melzack's fourth category is "miscellaneous." Here are some of his words:

Sensory: flickering, quivering, pulsing, throbbing, pounding, flashing, shooting, pricking, stabbing, cutting, pinching, pressing, gnawing, cramping, crushing, hot, burning, tingling, smarting, dull, aching, heavy.

Affective: exhausting, sickening, fearful, terrifying, gruelling, cruel, vicious, wretched, blinding.

Evaluative: annoying, troublesome, miserable, intense, unbearable.

Miscellaneous: tight, numb, penetrating, piercing, cool, cold, freezing, nagging, nauseating, torturing.

The McGill Pain Questionnaire, as it is called, provides doctors with a useful guide to what patients are experiencing. The sensory words can often assist in diagnosis; a patient's description of pain as throbbing or stabbing may give a clue to the disease or medical condition. If the questionnaire is repeated at an interval of days or weeks, insight is gained into the progress of a disease (or the course of recovery—for example, in postoperative pain). It must be borne in mind, of course, that the questionnaire produces a record of the patient's testimony, not an actual description of the pain. We all use words differently; some of us are inclined to minimize, others to exaggerate. (Although there are now versions of the McGill Questionnaire in several European languages, and also in Arabic and Japanese, translators are aware that few words have exact counterparts.)

On the basis of the questionnaire, Melzack worked out a scale running from 0 to 50. A pain described as mild is rated at 10, while a pain described as excruciating is rated at 40. It is (to repeat) an evaluation based on testimony, and its use does not imply that anyone is under the illusion that pain can be measured in the same way as temperature or loss of blood.

Our word *pain* comes from the French *peine*, the Latin *poena* and the Greek *poine*. The Greeks had several words for pain: *odyne* (from which we derive *anodyne*), *algos* (from which we

derive *analgesic*), *lype*, and *poine*. The meaning of *poine* changed
in classical Greek. First, it was the burden of inescapable hard
work ordained by the gods. In time, it became the prolonged
pain of battle wounds and of childbirth—pain with an ordained
purpose. Later, it came to mean punishment.

Our words *penalty* and *penalized* have the same root. In late
classical times, *poine* was applicable either to a punishment that
entailed physical injury, such as having a hand chopped off, or
to a punishment that did not, such as being banished. The
essential point was that something unpleasant was inflicted on
a person against his will. To this day, the pain that comes with
illness is often associated with the idea of punishment. Many a
sufferer has cried out, "What have I done to deserve this?"

Literature gives us more clues. It cannot have been a
strictly physical sensation that the dying Hamlet had in mind
when he pleaded with Horatio:

Absent thee from felicity awhile,
And in this harsh world draw thy breath in pain.
Hamlet, Shakespeare

Indeed, we often find pain linked with a variety of dis-
agreeable concepts, as in lines like these:

He has outsoared the shadow of our night;
Envy and calumny and hate and pain,
And that unrest which men miscall delight
Can touch him not and torture not again.
Adonais, Shelley

Doomed to go in company with pain,
And fear, and bloodshed, miserable train!
Character of the Happy Warrior, Wordsworth

In everyday speech, too, we use the word *pain* or the
adjective *painful* in ways that blur the distinction between the
physical and the mental or emotional. It is *painful* to be sepa-
rated from the person you love, and you are likely to *pine* (this
verb comes from the same root) for him or her. The illness or

death of the loved one is still more *painful*. Less tragically, it is *painful* to be defeated in an election, to be rejected for a job, or to get bad reviews for a book. To criticize a person sharply is to cause him *pain*—or, in phrases that embody obvious metaphors, to *hurt* him or *wound* him. And many a parent has exclaimed to an irritating child, "Why are you being such a *pain?*"

Were it possible to distinguish firmly between pain as a bodily process and pain as an emotional experience, there is little doubt that the English language would have produced noninterchangeable words to mark that distinction. As a matter of fact, our rich language does have a number of words with approximately the same meaning: *distress, anguish, suffering, misery, agony*. All of them, however, have the ambiguity—or, it might be better to say, the inclusive scope—that we have noted in the case of *pain*. A sprained ankle can be agony; trying to decide whether to end your marriage can also be agony.

These verbal usages point to something of central importance in the nature of the pain experience. Although the physical event related to the experience may, in many cases, be simple and obvious—the sprained ankle, the scalded hand—the experience itself cannot be reduced to that physical event. It is the human being who undergoes this experience; and a human being is an immensely complex organism with innumerable channels of interrelationship between what, for simplicity's sake, we call the body and the mind. Because each human being is unique and definably different from each other human being, it follows that the experience of pain is individual to that human being.

One of the authors (M.J.) has not previously been engaged in medical or scientific writing. When he told friends that he was collaborating on a book about pain, the most frequent response was "Do you mean physical or mental pain?" An important aim of this book is to dispel that dichotomy. There are physical and mental *causes* of pain: if a mountain climber has a fall, bruises and broken bones would be physical causes, while being left alone with no sign of a rescue party would be a mental cause. There are physical and mental *effects* of pain: weakness and high fever are physical, depression is mental. But pain itself cannot be either a purely physical or a purely mental experience.

The source of the confusion, to some extent, can be found in the fact that it is possible—quite usefully, and indeed with scientific accuracy—to describe and discuss pain with different vocabularies. The physiologist or neurologist will employ terms applicable to phenomena or changes in the body that are his concern. The psychologist will draw on a vocabulary appropriate to mental and emotional experiences. A mountain climber writing about his adventures would probably use both vocabularies and would thus help us to understand the unity of the physical and the mental.

In George Orwell's *1984*, O'Brien inflicts pain on Winston Smith (presumably, although Orwell does not make this explicit, through electric shocks) and says, "That was 40. You can see that the numbers on this dial run up to a hundred. . . . I have it in my power to inflict pain on you at any moment and to whatever degree I choose." This episode is highly effective in the framework of Orwell's imaginative novel, but it rests on an oversimplification. The dial could only register what O'Brien was doing; it could not register Smith's experience or reaction. The effect on Smith when the dial was at 40 might have been equivalent to the effect on another victim when the dial was at 30, or perhaps 50.

We now have, unfortunately, a great deal of evidence about torture by electric shock, employed by tyrannical regimes in many countries. Veterans of resistance movements recall with surprise that it was impossible to predict which individual would be able to hold out under torture. Sometimes, a leader known for his resolute character and his great physical strength was quickly broken; sometimes, a man or woman of retiring personality and slight physique held out indefinitely. We can say that some people are brave and others are not, and the differences are revealed only under stress. This statement is true enough in moral terms, but an equally true statement in scientific terms would be that, in the given situation, the two individuals varied in their tolerance of pain. One of them found it literally unbearable, while the other found the ability to bear it.

It is instructive to compare that experience with an experience familiar in normal life, namely, a visit to the dentist. You may come home and say, "It was agony," or even, "It was torture." However, there are crucial differences between the two experiences, of which you were aware while in the dentist's chair. The dentist is a friend, not an enemy. His activity is designed to benefit you, not to injure you, and you therefore have a positive motive for wishing him to continue and complete it. Moreover, if you do find the pain unbearable, you are free to ask him to stop or to give you an injection. All these factors will help you to be brave—in other words, to evaluate the pain as tolerable. But, although the dentist situation differs radically from the torture situation, it still cannot be precisely identical for two individuals or even for the same individual on two occasions. As well as the constant factors, there are variables affecting the perception of pain. These may include:

- The qualities of courage and moral strength that you possess, or that you believe you possess, or that you wish other people, including the dentist, to believe you possess
- Your sensitivity to the embarrassment of appearing cowardly or immature
- Your capacity for relaxation and freedom from tension, perhaps acquired in other contexts
- Your habitual tendency to anxiety and apprehension or, on the contrary, to optimism and confidence
- Your general state of health, and any adverse condition—a headache, sinus trouble, or perhaps a source of pain distant from your teeth—that may be affecting you when you arrive for your appointment

- Your recent experience of pain, if any
- Your state of happiness or unhappiness; a depressing experience in personal life or at work is likely to lower your morale and weaken your defenses
- Your past memories of dental treatment
- Your confidence, or lack of it, in this particular dentist

Can we now arrive at an answer to our question "What is pain?" We have seen that people have been struggling over the ages and in all languages to communicate the experience of a special form of misery called pain. In their desperation to communicate it, they have mixed cause and effect and have therefore used words such as "crushing" or "frightening." They have had recourse to analogies: "a stabbing pain" means "as though I were being stabbed." They have found language to be surprisingly inadequate to tell others about their inner feelings. Philosophers from Aristotle to Wittgenstein have struggled to translate the meaning of this crucial message.

Vernon Mountcastle, Professor of Physiology at Johns Hopkins, defined pain simply: "Pain is that sensory experience evoked by stimuli that injure or threaten to destroy tissue" (49). But is this a satisfactory definition? Harold Merskey, Professor of Psychiatry at the University of Western Ontario, called together a group of experienced and concerned people and they produced the following definition (46):

> Pain is an unpleasant sensory and emotional experience associated with actual or potential tissue damage, or described in terms of such damage.

They added crucial notes to this sentence:

> Pain is always subjective. Each individual learns the application of the word through experiences related to injury in early life. It is unquestionably a sensation in a part of the body but it is also always unpleasant and therefore also an emotional experience.

Many people report pain in the absence of tissue damage or any likely pathophysiological cause. Usually this happens for psychological reasons. There is no way to distinguish their experience from that due to tissue damage, if we take the subjective report. If they regard their experience as pain and if they report it in the same ways as pain caused by tissue damage, it should be accepted as pain. This definition avoids tying pain to the stimulus.

A final note refers to the nociceptor, a part of the body that registers injury:

Activity induced in the nociceptor and nociceptive pathways by a noxious stimulus is not pain, which is always a psychological state, even though we may well appreciate that pain most often has a proximate physical cause.

We shall use the word "pain" as it has been thus defined. It is a subtle definition in which each word and phrase is intentional and considered. Obviously, it applies only to adult humans and leaves open the question of what we can regard as pain in babies, animals, and those with whom we cannot communicate.

In this opening chapter, we hope to have clarified the distinction between the conditions giving rise to pain and the actual experience of pain. Medical knowledge enables us to state that certain classes of disease or injury are conducive to pain; it does not enable us to predict how much pain will be suffered by a particular man or woman in a particular time and place. This should be borne in mind as we go on, in the next chapter, to describe the—unfortunately, quite numerous—varieties of pain.

2

The Causes of Pain

All pains have causes. The most common cause is the presence of tissue that has been damaged by injury or disease. The brain must receive signals announcing the existence of such damage. These signals must also contain information about the location, extent, and nature of the damage. Here, we will first examine how these signals are generated in damaged tissue and transmitted to the brain and spinal cord.

INITIAL CAUSES

Aristotle understood that the senses were at the beginning of perception, and he used the word "incident" for what is perceived. British police stations maintain an incident room to which suspicious events are reported, and legal authorities everywhere employ the word "incident" for an occurrence that has not yet been examined. Their reason for this use of the word is that they wish to preserve pure observation separate from any assessment of meaning such as murder, suicide, or accident. The sensory nerve signals arising in damaged tissue are the data. "Data" means in English exactly what it means in Latin: that which is given. The data are not the meaning. The meaning is extracted from those data in the context of all other data. The injury signal is not the pain. However, because it may be crucial in triggering the pain, we will concentrate first on injury signals.

FROM PHILOSOPHY TO SCIENCE

While we repeatedly return to the hugely intelligent classical philosophers for education about ways of thinking, no one turns to their contemporaries to learn about mechanisms of thought and feeling. For 500 years after Aristotle, physiology was dominated by the Alexandrian school, whose lack of curiosity borders on silliness. For example, they maintained that blood vessels contain air. They were overthrown by Galen, who at least put blood in the blood vessels, but who dominated the next 1500 years of medicine with his humoral theory, in which the spirits of earth, air, fire, and water sloshed around in the body. We retain this fantasy nonsense in our language when we describe a person as cold-blooded, warm-hearted, or melancholic (Greek for having black bile). This model was not seriously questioned until the seventeenth century, when a natural philosophy began to question and observe. (See Fig. 1.)

René Descartes (1596–1650) was one of this new breed. He inspected the body by dissection as well as by introspection about what must be going on inside bodies. His intention was to give an anatomical location and physiological mechanism for Aristotelian sensation. This consisted of bundles of tiny filaments, the nerves, which ran from detectors in contact with the tissue through the spinal cord to a common sense center in the brain. We need not worry about the details, which were wrong but not bad guesses, considering the time. It is the idea which is important. The idea was that a relatively mechanical and reliable system reached from the structures that detected events on the periphery to the brain. Descartes described it thus:

> If, for example, fire comes near the foot, the minute particles
> of this fire, which as you know move with great velocity, have the

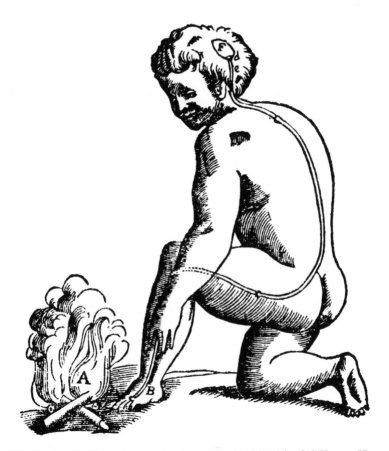

FIGURE 1. This illustration is taken from Descartes's 1644 book *L'Homme*. He proposed a signaling system that detects a stimulus and transmits the information to a sensory center (F). The message in the sensory center is read by a quite different system: the mind.

power to set in motion the spot of the skin of the foot which they touch, and by this means pulling upon the delicate thread which is attached to the spot of the skin, they open up at the same instant the pore against which the delicate thread ends, just as by pulling at one end of a rope one makes a bell which hangs at the other end to strike at the same instant.

We now know that this relatively mechanical signaling system runs only from the tissue to the spinal cord. These are the peripheral sensory fibers. Immediately on entering the spinal cord, the signals enter a gate control system, and a far more interesting and subtle process begins, rather than simply pulling on ropes and ringing bells.

FROM BELLS TO CELLS: DESCARTES TO CAJAL

The fundamental working units of the nervous system had been discovered by the beginning of this century. Santiago Ramon y Cajal (1852–1934) showed that the nervous system was not a diffuse interconnected network, but was made up of separate independent cells. This extraordinary man had his health wrecked while serving as a military doctor with the Spanish in Cuba. Returning to Spain, he settled on a gentler occupation, the study of anatomy, and exploited a newly discovered technique that revealed the shape of single cells. (See Fig. 2.)

This silver staining method had been discovered by the Italian Camillo Golgi (1843–1926). The two loathed each other

⎯⎯⎯⎯⎯⎯⎯⎯⎯⎯⎯⎯⎯⎯⎯⎯⎯⎯⎯⎯⎯⎯⎯⎯⎯⎯⎯▶

FIGURE 2. (A) Shape of the endings of three nerve fibers terminating among the cells of the spinal cord. These particular fibers originated in skin and delivered sensory signals about pressure on the skin. The horizontal line indicates 100 microns (4 thousandths of an inch). (B) Shape of a single cell in the spinal cord which receives messages by way of incoming fibers such as are shown in A. The horizontal line is 250 microns. (Courtesy of Drs. Clifford Woolf and Peter Shortland at University College, London, who had injected a dye into the individual nerve cells and fibers.)

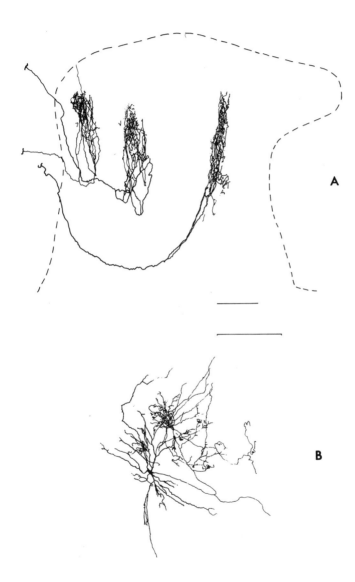

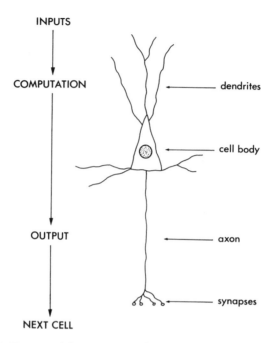

FIGURE 3. Diagram of the components found in all nerve cells. The arriving sensory signals end on the dendrites and on the cell body. The cell computes the consequence of the various inputs. It then generates an output that passes as nerve impulses along the axon. The axon terminates in synapses that are applied to the next cell.

because they came to opposite conclusions and refused to speak together even when they shared one of the first Nobel Prizes.

Our nervous systems are made up of hundreds of millions of separate cells, each with a special shape. It begins in the embryo as a simple spherical cell containing a nucleus within which are the genetic orders. This cell grows extensions, the dendrites, very like the branches of a tree, which collect the incoming signals (Fig. 3). The cell also puts out a long cylindri-

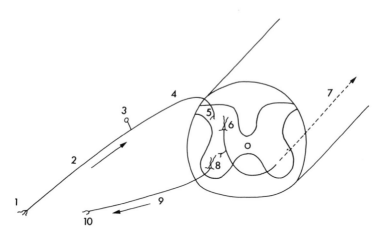

FIGURE 4. The input and output of the spinal cord. (1) Sensory nerve ending in tissue; (2) sensory fiber; (3) sensory nerve cell body: dorsal root ganglion cell (dorsal = toward the back); (4) dorsal root branch of the sensory fiber; (5) central terminal of the sensory fiber in the spinal cord; (6) nerve cell in the dorsal spinal cord that receives the sensory input; (7) axon of the nerve cell taking impulses to the brain; (8) nerve cell in the ventral (toward the abdomen) spinal cord; (9) axon of this cell leaving the cord in the ventral root; (10) termination of the axon on muscle where it causes contraction.

cal extension, the axon, which carries the outgoing signals. A special type of nerve cell is born, alongside the spinal cord. These sensory cells have no dendrites but grow out a single T-shaped axon. One branch of the T reaches out to the tissues, skin, muscle, and viscera. These axons are the sensory signaling fibers that carry nerve impulses from the peripheral tissues. They run in peripheral nerves such as the sciatic nerve (the major nerve of the leg). The other branch of the T grows into the spinal cord, where it makes contact with spinal cord cells (Fig. 4). This centrally running branch runs in a special bundle of such sensory fibers, the dorsal root, which enters the dorsal part of the spinal cord (dorsal means toward the back, and ventral means toward the front). Our sensory fibers can be up to 1 meter (3 ft, 3 in) long, for single sensory fibers run from the toes to the lower spinal cord. Some of these fibers, called A fibers, are relatively large in diameter, 2–12 microns (a micron is one-thousandth of a millimeter, and a millimeter is one twenty-fifth of an inch). A separate important group, C fibers, are relatively small, with a diameter of 0.25–1 micron.

DETECTION OF EVENTS BY SINGLE SENSORY NERVE FIBERS

The sensory end of the nerve fiber is sensitive to changes in its region, such as pressure or temperature, and to abnormal chemicals that leak from tissue when it is sick or damaged. If the disturbance is big enough, a sudden brief, explosive chemical event occurs in the nerve fiber. This all-or-none event is called a nerve impulse. The impulse, like the lighting of a fuse, sweeps along the nerve fiber and reaches the other end in the spinal cord. The impulse lasts only a thousandth of a second (a millisecond) and sweeps over the nerve fiber at 100 meters per second in the largest A fibers, but only 0.25 meter per second in the smallest C fibers. (Metric measurements are now generally used in scientific work, but we can give an idea of the speed by saying that it equals 225 miles per hour in the fastest fibers, but only a little more than half a mile per hour in the slowest.)

The bigger the event, the more nerve impulses per second are generated and transmitted. These nerve impulses, like Morse code dots, constitute the signal by which the peripheral nerve fibers inform the spinal cord of what has happened in the tissue. If they are prevented from traveling, no message is received; this is what happens when a dentist injects a local anesthetic. The nerve impulses generated in the sensory nerves in the teeth are blocked when they reach the part of the nerve soaked in local anesthetic, so that the brain receives no messages and the part of the face supplied by the blocked fibers feels numb.

Each single sensory fiber is special in two ways. First, it is interested only in its own target area. Second, it is interested only in particular events. The very large fibers are excited only by light pressure. Some fibers respond only to warming or to cooling. Some small myelinated fibers (that is, those enclosed in a substance called myelin) respond only to intense pressure; obviously these are of special importance with respect to pain. Many of the smallest fibers, the C fibers, respond to pressure, to high temperature (above 110 degrees Fahrenheit), and to abnormal chemicals. These fibers are clearly capable of signaling the presence of injury or sick tissue and are of particular interest to us. They are called nociceptors.

THE SIGNALS ENTER THE SPINAL CORD

As the sensory signals enter, they reach the end of the cell that has carried them and contact the first central cells at a junction, the synapse. The rules of communication across the synapse were established by Sir Charles Sherrington (1857–1952). They are never simple relay points. Here we encounter the first substantial deviation from Descartes, who shows his filaments as continuous from the periphery to deep in the brain. Sherrington showed that each synapse and cell was a computing, deciding, controlling area. Signals could be exaggerated, diminished, and merged even if they were operating simple reflexes. This gives us an understanding of the real biological point of the nervous system, which is not just a collection of puppet strings. For example, I. P. Pavlov (1849–1936), the Russian contemporary of Sherrington and Cajal, was showing that a sensory input (a bell) could take on a quite new effect or meaning if it was repeatedly associated with another sensory input (food). These conditioned reflexes show that the entering signals are not just under control, but enter a modifiable dynamic system, in which the outcome is not the simple consequence of the second-by-second input. We are at the beginning of a farewell ceremony for Descartes. Later, we shall explain how the process of selection and calculation begins immediately at the entry point—the gate.

Thanks to remarkable work carried out in Sweden, we now know precisely which input signals arrive at the spinal cord (67). It was found to be possible to insert very fine tungsten needles painlessly into peripheral nerves and to record the single sensory nerve impulses on their way from the periphery to the spinal cord. While recording the input signal, we can ask the person involved to say what he felt. We are, in fact, asking what has happened and what will happen.

A very exact lawful relationship can be worked out for the answer to the question "What has happened?" The nature of the stimulus has been encoded as nerve signals. In the case of injury, that process is called nociception. The answer to the question "What will happen?" is not completely dependent on the input nerve signals. Those signals will now enter the central nervous system across synapses where they can interact with past events, ongoing events, and intentions. The laws of these interactions determine the consequence of the arriving signal and the nature of pain. We can now begin to describe the actual consequences of disease and tissue damage as a cause of pain, knowing that the existence of damage and of peripheral signals will not have a simple direct effect in terms of pain.

A SCRATCH

By examining the course of events in a trivial injury, we can learn a lot about more serious injuries involving pain. Try the experiment of inflicting a scratch on your arm. Press your thumbnail into a spot near the wrist until it hurts; then drag your nail rapidly along the skin toward your elbow, keeping the pressure constant. Now, feel and look.

Immediately after the scratch, you see a white line on the skin. This means that the blood vessels have clamped down in direct reaction to the injury. Some seconds later, the scratch turns red and this red mark slowly broadens. This is not bleeding; it is a dilation of the blood vessels produced by chemicals leaking into the tissue. After several minutes, the mark shrinks again and you are left with a quite precise, bright red line on your skin. Examining this line in a good slanting light, you can see a shiny swelling, or weal. This indicates that the blood vessels are leaking fluid into the damaged skin. During this time, you may have felt a slight burning along the scratch, and you also observe a prickly feeling if you run your fingers lightly across the scratch. The reason for these sensations is that the nerves have been sensitized by chemicals released by the damaged tissue.

You have now produced the four classical signs of inflammation:

1. Redness, caused by dilation of the blood vessels.
2. Heat, caused in the first place by a flow of warm blood brought by the dilated blood vessels. If the damage is extensive and prolonged, the brain will respond to it by producing a fever, with flushing, high temperature, and sweating. Nerve impulses are also interpreted as a feeling of burning, so that the affected area feels hotter than it is.
3. Swelling, produced by fluid moving from the blood into the area of damage. In severe injuries this loss of fluid is dangerous; this is why rescue workers and hospitals use saline bottles to top up the blood volume.
4. Pain, occurring in three stages. First, there is the cutting pain you felt while the damage was in progress, then the burning pain left by the damage, and finally, the lingering tenderness.

With regard to pain, this experiment teaches two important lessons. One is that the pain was always bearable because it was self-inflicted and you were in control; you did not, for example, press too hard with your thumbnail. If someone else had scratched you in the same way, the sensation would have been quite different. The pain would have been far more intense and would have had frightening, threatening aspects. Later, in discussing what can be done to help people in pain—and how they can help themselves—we shall see that they can change and limit the experience of pain by establishing a sense of control.

The other lesson is related to our observation of three different kinds of pain, occurring in sequence. Pain is not a single phenomenon; it takes various forms, each with its own descriptive vocabulary and its own implications. The later pains mentioned above (the burning pain and the subsequent tenderness) were caused partly by new nerve impulses generated in the damaged tissue, partly because nerve cells in the brain and the spinal cord were alerted by the injury, with the result that they overreacted to even the smallest messages from the damaged tissue.

The first, instantaneous pain and the later pains had different meanings. The first pain signaled the need to arrest or limit the damage—"don't go on scratching, don't scratch too hard or too deep." The later pains announced that the damage was over and the process of recovery could begin, given the existence of suitable conditions—"don't touch your arm again." We tend to think that all pain is the same, distinguished only by the gradations of "big" or "small," "bad" or "not so bad." But these distinctions in meaning can be just as important.

A TWISTED ANKLE

This common experience is worth a thoughtful analysis. Typically, you feel a flash of pain—sudden, sharp, and precisely localized. It dies down almost as quickly as it appeared. The sequel is a quite different pain—deep, dull, and spreading. This tells you that you will be in trouble the next day, and probably next week. When joints and tendons are damaged, even slightly, they set off a train of nervous events that serve to optimize the recovery process. Sensations of tenderness and aching are not confined to the area of damage, but spread over the foot and the lower leg. You have to limp; your limping prevents full movement of the damaged ankle and thus creates good conditions for recovery. You may well be able to find a position in which your ankle hurts only slightly or not at all. From this, you can deduce that there is no constant generator of pain. However, if you move your ankle or make your foot bear pressure, the pain will recur. The injury has caused the nervous system to lower its threshold so that pain is triggered by a normally innocuous movement. The ankle is working at reconstructing itself by building new tissue, and this fragile tissue could be disrupted by ordinary exertion.

TOOTHACHE

The human face, lips, tongue, and teeth are exquisitely sensitive, being heavily and specially innervated. When things go wrong, they can become a minefield. There are no nerves in the enamel that protects a tooth, but plenty of nerve endings in the bony substance (dentin) underneath. If the enamel is cracked or decayed to expose the dentin, sharp and very nasty pains can be set off, especially by food that is very hot, very cold, sweet, or sour. Pain in the teeth, unlike pain in the skin, is often inaccurately localized; the sufferer may point to the lower jaw when the problem is really in the upper jaw. When back teeth are involved, the pain often seems to be an earache. When pain is located at a distance from the diseased tissue, it is called "referred pain." This is very common when deep tissue is affected. Disorders of the heart, gut, uterus, and joints all show predictable repeated patterns of pain far removed from the problem. These patterns are a diagnostic challenge. They are the consequence of the convergence of different types of sensory afferents on first central cells. We will be able to use them as an example of the nature of central processing of arriving sensory signals. Nor is there any correlation between the amount of tissue damage and the intensity of the pain.

If the disease spreads into the soft pulp of the tooth, the pain changes its character; it is severe, generally throbbing, and long-lasting. It radiates so that it appears to be affecting the ear, the temple, or the cheek. Yet it may suddenly abate, even though the disease is relentlessly progressing. A dentist needs to be skillful to make a correct diagnosis when the patient's senses are producing inaccurate information. The truth is that pain is a very poor reporting system. After a night made miserable by toothache, you may feel in the morning that the pain has gone and cancel your appointment with the dentist, although the disease or decay is as much of a reality as ever. The doctrine that pain is a useful signal needs heavy qualification.

SUDDEN INJURY

An acute injury produces a barrage of nerve impulses in the sensory nerve fibers. Localized damage, such as the insertion of a hypodermic needle, will fire off a small number of nerve fibers. There are fewer nerve fibers in a given area of the upper arm than in the tips of the fingers. Therefore, the same needle pushed into a fingertip produces activity in more fibers than if it is pushed into the shoulder. Hitting your thumb with a hammer stimulates a higher-frequency barrage in single fibers and stimulates a large number of fibers. Generation of these injury signals is inevitable and predictable, depending on the location and intensity of the injury and on the type of injury (for example, mechanical, chemical, or a burn).

The inevitable injury signal now enters the spinal cord, and most people would predict that pain is equally inevitable. This prediction is so crucial that we devote a special chapter to it, because it involves one of the most important issues about the nature of pain. In the present context, the relevant point is that pain has its own time course, which is not necessarily the same as the time course of injury. Most doctors and nurses can tell stories of people who injured themselves—sometimes quite seriously—but didn't realize it until another person informed them of it, or until they noticed blood dripping onto the floor. One recorded example is that of a linoleum layer who cut his finger with a sharp blade, so that about an inch of fingertip remained attached only by a narrow flap of skin. Astonished that he was feeling no pain, he washed and bandaged his finger and drove in his car to the hospital. On the way, he felt hot throbbing sensations, and by the time he entered the emergency clinic, he was in pain. But at the time when he was still pain-free, he was fully aware of what had happened and his injury-detecting sensory fibers were sending their messages at maximum intensity.

POSTOPERATIVE PAIN

Surgical operations necessarily result in tissue damage, but there are crucial differences between these injuries and accidental injuries, which allow us to consider the relationship of injury to pain. In the first place, it is crucial that these "injuries" are requested by the patient with the overall intention of benefit. The patient is prepared and reassured and is in capable hands. During the act of tissue damage, the patient is unaware, either because he is under general anesthesia or because local anesthesia has blocked the arriving injury signals. On waking up, most patients are soon in pain. In a study of pain in 514 patients who had orthopedic operations under general anesthesia, 56% needed analgesia within the first two hours (39). However, as in all other painful states, there is a wide variability. Five percent of the patients never required analgesia during the whole recovery period.

The pain has a time course not only in intensity, but in

nature and quality, moving from acute to more long term. Since operations—like many injuries—go deep, there is a variety of pains, each with its rules and distinct natural history. For example, women who have had a cesarean section report at least three separate recognizable pains. First, there is the incision, with its stitches, as an obvious source. Next, surprisingly, these mothers report painful uterine contraction pains exactly the same as those of mothers who have given birth vaginally. Finally, there are deep pelvic and abdominal pains which come and go and are difficult to describe. Since, as Hippocrates noted in one of his aphorisms, one pain beats out another, the mother reports sometimes one pain and sometimes another and sometimes a period of blissful relief. The injury to her tissue is stable and so are the injury signals, but the brain interprets the situation in a variable exploratory fashion. The shifting nature of the pains adds to the patient's misery since she may take them as disaster signals.

The most obvious difference between surgery and accident is that the injury is not only intentional, but is planned. This provides time for preparation. The patient's natural fear of the unknown can be at least partially alleviated by explanation, and even the briefest of discussions with the anesthesiologist has been shown to reduce postoperative pain. In China, it is the custom to admit surgical patients days before their operations. They busy themselves on the wards sweeping up and serving meals. In the process, they become familiar not only with the staff, but with postoperative patients who turn out not to be suffering nearly so badly as the future victim feared. This method works wonders. Unfortunately, it is not available to Western patients, who are lucky if they spend an hour in bed in a high-tech hospital before being whisked off to the operating theater.

The most exciting possibilities for preparation are yet to come. It is possible that postoperative pain may be prevented rather than treated when it occurs. Rather simple application of these principles can increase the number of those who never complain of pain from 5% to 15% and delay the need for a first analgesic by between 2 and 9 hours.

BURNS

Some 80,000 people are hospitalized each year in America with burns or scalds (14). Burns produce pains as severe and prolonged as any. At the instant of burning, the amount of pain varies from one individual to another and is influenced by circumstances. It then settles down to a relatively constant level, though movement makes it worse. Sadly, it is exacerbated by necessary therapeutic procedures, such as changes of dressings, topical medicines, and skin grafts. As healing proceeds, actual pain is gradually replaced by intense tingling and itching. Like almost all pains, burn pains vary at different times of the day and night, although the state of injury or recovery is of course unaffected by the clock.

As time passes and regenerative tissue grows, patients often become more and more uncomfortable and unhappy. Various explanations are possible. It could be that nerves are regrowing in the burned parts of the body and are therefore able to report the presence of abnormal tissue to the brain. The pain may also be an effect of accumulating exhaustion and sleeplessness in the isolated sterile atmosphere in which the patient is kept to reduce contact with the burn—an ordeal likely to test the most stoical person. What can be said is that this pain cannot be a useful signal at the time and is indeed utterly useless, since the damage is perfectly obvious both to the sufferer and to the doctors. Nor is there any reliable correlation between the severity of the pain and the depth or location of the burn.

The pain endured by the burned is inevitably intensified by their (justified) anxiety regarding the prospects of full recovery. Reassurance would seem desirable, but the unfortunate truth is that the world's greatest experts cannot yet guarantee that the burns will heal without scars, or that there will be no residual infection. Gradually, however, the situation is becoming less gruesome. By attacking the multiple problems as a whole rather than singly, and by making use of the essential help of the patient, ways are being found to deal with what had been seen as the unavoidable consequences of burns.

HEART ATTACK

William Heberden, writing in 1768, originated the term *angina pectoris*—literally, anguish of the chest—to designate "a very distinctive disorder of the chest attended with a sense of strangling and anxiety." He stressed that it was often accompanied by *angor animi*—anguish of the mind. The early physicians were almost as confused and frightened as their patients, for they did not know what was happening, but knew that it was bad. We now know that angina occurs when an area in the heart has an inadequate blood supply. This can happen suddenly and catastrophically if one of the major arteries to the heart is blocked by a blood clot. More usually, there is a slow closing over of the arteries, which gradually narrow and supply less and less blood. A person to whom this happens is in no pain when at rest, but once he exerts himself, the heart must work harder to pump blood around the body, and a point is reached when the narrowed arteries cannot supply enough to meet the demand. The heart muscle then generates nerve impulses announcing an inadequate flow of blood, and the person experiences angina of effort. This condition may be remedied by the coronary bypass operation, in which new blood vessels are sewn into place to bypass the blocked or constricted arteries. A similar condition can occur in the legs: arteries gradually get blocked, the blood supply fails to meet the demand when the legs are used for walking, and the result is pain. This condition is called intermittent claudication.

A heart attack, or in medical language a myocardial infarction, is the sudden blocking of an artery to the heart muscle. What does it feel like? Often the first signs are breathlessness, a vague feeling of discomfort in the chest, and unpleasant gastric sensations resembling those of indigestion. When President Eisenhower suffered his first heart attack, he fooled both himself and his doctors and was sent to bed with an antacid to settle his stomach. But, after a while, a deep pain develops and lasts for minutes or hours. Patients cannot give a definite location for this pain; they speak of pressing, squeezing, or "a band round the chest." At this stage there may well be nausea, vomiting, and profuse sweating. Quite possibly, the patient gasps, "I'm dying"—and believes it. But Eisenhower, for one, completed his two terms as President and enjoyed several years of retirement.

During the transition period, the pain appears to move from the depths and settle in the chest wall. The left arm begins to feel strangely numb or cramped, and the pain moves to involve the arm and hand. It may also radiate into the neck and jaw. By this time, most patients will have received morphine, which provides very satisfying relief both for the pain and for the anguish.

Many heart attacks develop more slowly than this and are therefore less dramatic and frightening, but the characteristics are the same—the pain in the chest, and the later referred pain in the left arm. This referred pain is not a delusion. It is a real event; the whole arm from shoulder to hand is weak and tender.

All this sounds quite simple, and the pathology seems highly specific. But diseases of the stomach, the aorta, or the gallbladder can produce pains very similar to those of a heart attack, so the skilled physician will be cautious in his interpretation of the complaints. He has to make the correct differential diagnosis although the pains are changing in their nature as time passes and the clues they give are wildly misleading. If the doctor has diagnostic problems, what about the anxious, terrified person to whom all this is happening? He is short of breath, he is sweating, his heart is pounding, and he has a strange pain in the chest. Not surprisingly, to be sure of getting adequate help, he says that he's having a heart attack. To make an investigation and assure him that there's nothing wrong with his heart may not be good enough. He may be wrong about the heart attack, but he is right in knowing that there is trouble somewhere. And it's a sound rule that there must be something wrong with anyone who is in pain.

Let us consider three aspects of the pain during a heart attack: its time course, its location, and its intensity. From observing patients in intensive care units, we know that the episode can begin with the sudden blocking of a major blood vessel. Within seconds, the nerves in the region deprived of blood are sending a maximal barrage of nerve impulses to the brain and the spinal cord. This barrage is associated with reactions of alarm and nausea and with a general feeling that something is wrong. The nerve impulses that have entered the spinal cord also trigger a slow rise of excitability in all the nearby nerve cells. Even though the input signals die down, they have sparked off a spreading fire of excitability. The normal function of the nerve cells is to transmit detailed and precise information about events on the skin and in the muscles, of which we are consciously aware. Therefore, when such cells are excited, our consciousness places the origin of the problem in skin or muscle. Furthermore, since these cells have become more sensitized than usual, they interpret a real input signal from the arm or chest as being painful even if the actual event was a gentle pressure. Thus, a brief, abrupt alarm signal originating in deep tissue (in the heart) has set off reactions in that part of the nervous system with which we have only the vaguest conscious sensory contact, because it deals with internal organs. As the effect spreads to nerve cells concerned with skin and muscle, we seem to be getting signals from parts of the body with which we have detailed and accurate conscious contact, as well as a vocabulary to talk about them. This is why the person undergoing the heart attack describes and remembers it in terms of the "wrong" area.

The most bizarre referred pain effects occur in the case of some liver diseases, which are felt as pain and tenderness in the shoulder. The explanation is this: while an infant is developing in the womb, some tissue in the embryo migrates from the shoulder region to make the diaphragm and takes its nerve supply along with it. If the diaphragm is inflamed, it sends nerve impulses to the shoulder area of the spinal cord. The increased excitability then spreads to cells that receive information from the real shoulder. The patient is sure that the pain, and its source, are in the shoulder—and who can blame him?

We have seen, then, that the time course and location of pain fail to match the actual events. This may not be disastrous, since adequate knowledge enables us to make the right interpretation. What about the intensity of pain? Readers will know by this time that the apparently common-sense rule of "the worse the damage, the more pain" is far from reliable. To follow this rule in the case of heart attacks would indeed be disastrous.

Silent heart attacks, in which pain gives no indication of coronary disease, have been known since they were described by Sir William Osler in 1910. With the invention of the electrocardiogram and, later, more sophisticated ways of measuring the heart's circulation, it has become much easier to detect this silent myocardial ischemia (12). But about 600,000 people each year die of ischemic heart disease in the United States, many of them suddenly and without previous symptoms.

Examination of middle-aged men shows three groups with signs of clearly inadequate blood supply but no pain. The first group (one to three million people in North America) has no symptoms and no history of angina or of myocardial infarction. The second group has had heart attacks and appear to have recovered. The third group has episodes of angina and can be shown to have silent episodes of insufficient blood flow between the angina episodes. It is evident that there is a large detectable background to predictable catastrophic episodes. It will not, therefore, surprise American readers that a patient in California has already successfully sued his physician for half a million dollars for failing to screen for silent ischemia. The man had several risk factors for coronary disease: he was middle-aged, male, drinking, smoking, and overweight, with little exercise. Six months before suffering a heart attack, he had visited his doctor, with the complaint of influenza. He claimed his doctor should have taken the opportunity to screen him. Unfortunately, we cannot sue our own sensory systems for failing to announce the presence of ischemia. In a study of 7599 ischemic episodes, only 32% were painful. This failure of our sensory system is lethal because the disasters are preventable and, even when they occur, treatable if immediate medication with new drugs is given.

This is an important conclusion, not only for heart disease, but for pain in general. When a patient who has suffered a severe heart attack is hospitalized, it often turns out that he had an earlier attack, which he dismissed as not worth mentioning, certainly not worth complaining about. As a system for reporting damage, pain can only be rated as inefficient and sloppy. The practical lessons are that health professionals should pay close attention to all complaints of pain, even when described as trivial, and that we should all pay attention to the sloppy reports delivered by our nervous systems.

PERSISTENT PAINS: OSTEOARTHRITIS

We turn now to a consideration of types of pain that persist for a long time—perhaps for years, perhaps until death. Pain of this kind is described as chronic (from the Greek *chronos*, time). Chronic pains have the same characteristics as acute pains, and other characteristics too.

Osteoarthritis (often referred to simply as arthritis) is the most common rheumatic disease, causing pain and disability in many elderly people. What happens is an erosion of the cartilage of a joint, such as the hip, knee, or wrist. The bone near the joint is forced to reorganize, and swelling occurs outside the joint. When the condition is advanced, some victims of osteoarthritis experience severe, intractable pain, but others have little or none. The disease is likely to set in—at first, insidiously and in a small way—around the age of 50. By the age of 75, 85% of people have signs of osteoarthritis. Arthritis of the knees and hands is two-and-a-half times more common in women than in men, but arthritis of the hips affects the sexes equally.

What is it like to suffer from osteoarthritis? In the early stages, you feel an unpleasant aching, but you can relieve it by movement and massage. At a more advanced stage, movement and weight bearing make the pain worse. Given that some activity is inevitable during the day, the pain is at its worst in the evening. Gradually, you attempt less and less movement and activity, and so become capable of less. Another development is a painful morning stiffness, with sensations of referred pain at some distance from the affected joint. This referred pain makes movement yet more difficult; thus, if you have a painful shoulder, you may also have a clumsy hand. Other problems are diminishing mobility and exhaustion from disturbed sleep. Few homes, rich or poor, have chairs suitable for an arthritic person. Settling yourself into the average chair is painful because it involves weight bearing on arthritic joints during the descent. Once you are in a low chair, your joints are overflexed beyond their comfortable range, even limited movement is difficult, and stiffness sets in. If you stay in your chair and watch television, the program is certain to show young people breakdancing.

Millions of people resign themselves stoically to this wretched condition, accepting it as the inevitable consequence of growing old. They have long since stopped complaining to doctors or relatives, as there is clearly nothing to be done about it. Yet other people are celebrating their eightieth birthday by playing tennis or going for a swim.

The strange fact is that we don't understand why people with arthritis are in such pain. The obvious tissue damage is in structures that contain no nerves. Adjacent tissue is secondarily affected, and therapy aimed at this tissue can be quite success-ful and is more practical than complete replacement of the joint by surgery. The most puzzling aspect of the situation is that some people whose joints have suffered gross destruction are limited in movement but are not in pain. Again, injury and pain fail to keep step. It follows that we must try to deal with pain as a problem in itself, instead of accepting it as the natural accom-paniment of old age—or even of osteoarthritis.

The trouble is that the disease itself, the immobility, the pain, and the attitudes of the victim and of other people are interacting complications. The disease produces pain, which worsens the immobility, which intensifies the disease. The victim becomes sadder and more depressed, alienating those who might be willing to offer help. Osteoarthritis robs us of the freedom and independence we won as we advanced into adult life from the restraints of childhood—no wonder it is hard to bear.

RHEUMATOID ARTHRITIS

This condition, also regrettably widespread, differs from osteoarthritis in that it can occur at any age, even in childhood or youth. It is seen in 2.5% of the population, with 0.2% having persistent disease. The long-term outlook is good in many cases, but it's hell while it lasts. The most obvious symptoms are in the joints, particularly the hands, but they are part of a general disease; the patient may feel feverish, weak, and gener-ally unwell. Rheumatoid arthritis tends to affect many joints at the same time, but the worst affected are usually fingers and toes.

The onset can be quite insidious. The first signs are swell-ing of soft tissue, stiffness, and pain. Typically, the swelling is worst in the early morning and improves with activity during the day, but many patients develop further symptoms when they get tired in the evening. The joints become swollen and very tender, and there is a surprisingly rapid wasting of the nearby muscles. These symptoms die down in time, but if destruction of the joints has gone too far, it leads to deformity and loss of function. We have all seen people with distorted, spindly fingers swollen at their base; this is the long-term result of a severe attack, and the main problem is that the fingers are frozen rigid.

During the acute phase of the disease, pain arises from inflammation and also from the general feeling of being weak and below par. Apathy and pain are close companions on the road to the slough of despond. To say, "Cheer up!" to a person with rheumatoid arthritis is useless, indeed cruel. Disease and pain, between them, produce a condition very like depression. The signs of this condition are reluctance to attempt movement, loss of appetite, constipation, loss of weight, poor sleep—and a loathing for bright, cheerful chatter.

Friends and relatives of sufferers from this disease are in a dilemma. To insist on effort and movement seems wrong; a broken leg heals best when immobile, and the same should be true of a weakened body. When a dog feels sick, it lies down and snaps at its owner if he tries to force it to go for a walk. Why shouldn't a human being behave like this too? This logic appears sensible, yet there is a weight of evidence that passive inactivity makes the disease and the pain worse. In a later chapter, we shall discuss this problem more fully.

CANCER

There are only two good things to be said about cancer. One: some cancers are curable. Two: not all cancers are painful. Admittedly, most cancers are painful at some stage, but today the pain can be controlled in a highly satisfactory way. What worries most people is not death, but the manner of dying; the prospect of agonizing pain, total dependence, and loss of dignity arouses a natural horror.

By its very nature, cancer is insidious. Cancerous cells are 99% the same as the normal cells from which they arise; the 1% difference is in their ability to divide and multiply. As they grow, they are accepted as normal by their neighbors, which fail to notice the difference. When the body recognizes an alien presence—such as a bacterium, a piece of dirt, or a smashed cell—the reaction is inflammation, accompanied by pain. But because a cancer cell does not appear to be alien, no such reaction occurs.

Initially, the cancer cells multiply in one place to form a lump, known as the primary tumor. Sometimes the cells of this tumor divide at a slow pace and stay close to the original site without infiltrating any other body structures. In this case, although the cells are cancerous they are not malignant and the tumor is described as a benign growth. When it is removed, the body is out of danger. Sometimes, however, the cancer cells push aside their normal neighbors, break away from the primary tumor, enter lymph channels or blood vessels, and start a new colony—a secondary tumor or metastasis—at a distance. The faster the cancerous cells divide, and the more they infiltrate and colonize, the more malignant is the cancer. Each secondary tumor, following the example of the primary tumor, grows wherever it has settled.

Throughout the entire period of this initial development, the cancer victim feels no pain. This is why it is advisable to take note and inform a doctor whenever you observe a lump—and a painless lump needs particular attention. Pain in cancer is a late sign, which tells us that the cancer is dangerously advanced. It indicates that the tumor has grown to the point where its very size has a mechanical effect. When this happens will depend on the location of the tumor. It may be growing in relatively free space where it can expand without causing pressure or destruction. If its expansion is restricted, it will press on tissue and destroy normal cells. The first signs of trouble may be caused by the closing of a channel, such as a blood vessel, a lung bronchus, or the gastrointestinal tract. The attack on normal cells sets off an inflammatory reaction, and this is painful. Bone, in particular, is a structure whose rigidity forms a barrier to expansion. Consequently, bone pain is common, but in its early stages it responds to ordinary anti-inflammatory drugs.

The bone pains are not produced by the cancer itself, but by the secondary effects of the cancer on normal tissue. It can, for instance, weaken the bone so much that it collapses and breaks. If the fracture involves normal bone structure, it causes pain like any other fracture; if it involves only the cancerous part of the bone, it causes no pain. Once we grasp the fact that the cancer itself is not painful, we can understand why some cancer victims die without experiencing any pain at all.

An understanding of the mechanism of cancer pain is important for two reasons. It demonstrates yet again (perhaps we should apologize for repeating this so often in different contexts) that pain is an inefficient reporting system. The cancer sufferer has every right to be angry at his pain, for it did not act as an early warning and it contributes nothing toward recovery. It is, in fact, absolutely useless.

Second, given that the cause of the pain is the destruction of normal tissue, it follows that cancer pain is no different from any other pain—from the pain caused by some other disease or by accidental injury. It is, therefore, right and necessary to do everything we can to reduce the pain. The future for the cancer patient may involve surgery, chemotherapy, or radiotherapy, each of which is something of an ordeal. Moreover, death is always at least a possibility. Pain merely makes it harder to face this future calmly and with courage. Even terminal cancer patients have a right to live in the true sense of the word—to feel normal emotions, to think rationally, to make decisions—until they die. If that is the aim, pain is nothing but an unwelcome intrusion.

As cancers expand and produce painful secondary effects, they may be doing so in particularly fragile areas. Tiny tumors in the cerebral cortex can do enough damage to cause epilepsy.

In other parts of the brain, they can block the channel draining fluid from the brain, and the consequent rise in pressure causes headaches. These events may warn the physician that the cancer has reached a danger point, but that is no reason not to deal with the immediate problem—for example, by installing a new drainage duct to bypass the blocked channel.

Finally, cancer pains themselves have further effects. They often set off muscle contractions that cause cramps, lingering aches, and tenderness in regions deep in the body tissue. One consequence is to make movement difficult; the patient may be able to find a comfortable position, but may be unable to move out of it. Cancer can also infiltrate and damage nerves. This produces special problems and leads us into the general subject of nerve damage.

PERIPHERAL NERVE DAMAGE

Bundles of nerve fibers combine to form large nerves, such as the sciatic nerve in the leg and the ulnar nerve in the arm. Sensory nerve fibers, carrying sensory impulses, pass through "portholes" between the vertebrae—called foramina—and form the spinal roots. These, in turn, enter the spinal cord. Similar nerve fibers originating in the face and mouth group together to form the trigeminal nerve. It forms a root that enters the lower part of the brain stem.

If a nerve is cut by injury or disease, the area it serves becomes numb or anesthetized because the sensory nerve can no longer carry impulses from the tissue to the spinal cord (see 1, 2, 3, and 4 in Fig. 4). Nerves also contain motor fibers—distinct from sensory fibers—which carry impulses from the cord to muscles (9 and 10 in Fig. 4) and are necessary for movement. Thus, when nerves are cut, the area they supply is numb and paralyzed. The spinal cord reacts to the loss of arriving sensory signals and increases its excitability to such a level that a very unpleasant pain can develop in the numb area.

Nerve damage can also develop slowly when nerve fibers are selectively infected by a virus. Shingles is an infection of the sensory, not the motor, nerves, having the effect of a skin eruption, a burning pain, and extreme tenderness. The viral damage completely destroys some nerve fibers and leaves others in an abnormal state. Shingles is caused by an explosion of virus duplication affecting a bundle of fibers supplying a single nerve root. Therefore, it produces a painful rash running in a strip from back to front in an area served by one fraction of all the body nerves. On the face, it attacks one of the three divisions of the trigeminal nerve; most often, this is the division that supplies the forehead, so that inflammation and pain occur on one side of the forehead and on the eyelids, but not on the rest of the face.

Bacteria can also destroy nerves, with painful consequences. The most dramatic is syphilis, which can attack the sensory roots to produce *tabes dorsalis*, a very serious condition, characterized by shooting pains and feelings of numbness and leading to the destruction of large nerve fibers in the sensory roots. Today this stage of syphilis is forestalled by penicillin, but Baroness Blixen (the writer Izak Dinesen, author of *Out of Africa*) lived too long ago to benefit by it and described the "lightning pains" and "numbing cramps" of tabetic crisis.

Thus, painful nerve damage can result from bacterial infection, from trauma, from viruses, and from metabolic diseases. The most common of the latter are alcoholism and diabetes. The last years of President Nasser's life were spent with numbed, tingling, agonizingly painful limbs, and his frequent absences from Egypt were caused by fruitless attempts to find relief from his diabetic neuropathy.

In all cases of nerve damage—rapid or slow, caused by a virus or by cancer—one effect may be a very unpleasant form of pain called deafferentation pain. The afferent nerves are those which bring sensory information to the brain and spinal cord, and their interruption is called deafferentation. Nerves that carry impulses *from* the brain and spinal cord to peripheral tissue are the efferent nerves, or motor nerves. Most nerves are a bundle of afferent and efferent nerve fibers, conveying information in one direction and motor signals in the other. One of the worst aspects of these deafferentation pains is that they are not relieved by analgesics, which warns us that their mechanism must differ from that of most pains.

If a large nerve is suddenly cut or blocked, one effect is an illusion that feeling still exists in the part that has been anesthetized (deprived of feeling). Almost all of us have had this experience in the dentist's chair. When a dentist injects a local anesthetic, he has introduced a blocking agent into branches of the trigeminal nerve that carry sensory nerve impulses from the face and the mouth to the brain. He selects the nerves that supply one side of either the upper or the lower jaw. The patient feels numbness and is paralyzed in that lip. Afterward, the lip is still numb but seems to be larger than life; the patient is under the illusion that he has a swollen lip. The lip is paralyzed as well as anesthetized because the local anesthetic has blocked both the sensory and the motor fibers. After a while, the drug is washed away by the bloodstream and normal feeling— including tenderness if a tooth has been extracted—returns.

For the amputee, there is no such easy return to normal. The cutting of the nerves has deprived the brain of the customary trickle of innocuous sensory impulses from the periphery. The brain is alerted to this distortion of the normal input and gives special attention to the missing limb. It is impossible for the brain to accept such a change passively; it issues a steady stream of commands to explore and investigate the novel situation.

When a nerve is violently damaged by injury or disease, it generates an emergency barrage of impulses, called the injury discharge. This brief alarm signal rapidly dies down, but the impulses have entered the central nervous system, where they trigger long-lasting effects of the kind we described following a twisted ankle. Nor is this all. Unlike telephone wires, nerve fibers are alive. When cut, they attempt to regenerate by putting out fine sprouts that reach into the tissue that has been deprived of its nerve supply. These sprouts, like other immature forms of life, are noisy and unstable, by which we mean that they generate impulses without any provocation and are very easily stimulated by slight pressure. They also become sensitive to chemicals, especially those emitted by the sympathetic nervous system. It should be explained here that there are two efferent motor systems. One drives the muscles and produces movement. The other, called the autonomic system, regulates all other tissues; it governs the blood vessels, the sweat glands, and the glands of the heart, the lungs, and all internal organs. It is divided into the sympathetic and the parasympathetic systems. Sympathetic nerve fibers emit a chemical called norepinephrine, which excites damaged nerves.

Nerve damage is responsible for another, gradual process. Nerve fibers are extensions of a nerve cell body (see Fig. 3). The cell body manufactures the materials needed for the growth and maintenance of the fibers. A system like a conveyor belt takes this material to the periphery. On its return journey, it picks up chemicals found in the periphery. If there has been damage in the periphery, there will have been changes in these chemicals, and the cell body will recognize and react to these changes. As the chemicals enter the nervous system, further changes are produced. Thus, nerve damage has two kinds of consequence—rapid changes triggered by nerve impulses (described above) and these slower changes induced by chemicals.

What this means for the patient is a deafferentation syndrome. A continuous prickling or burning pain is generated, either by impulses from damaged nerves or by intensely alerted nerve cells. Moreover, because the cells are highly excitable, even impulses from undamaged nerves set off an explosion of activity, and a light, harmless stimulus causes a stab of intense pain.

A pain deriving from nerve damage is always individual; no two people will have exactly the same experience. However, certain generalizations can be made. The pain always has a time sequence, with an acute emergency phase and a later prolonged phase. Pains of deep origin have a component referring to distant structures. Tenderness is particularly troublesome, because an apparently harmless contact or movement can give rise to serious pain. Finally—once again!—there may be no logical relationship between the amount of damage and the amount of pain. Hence, we should not be astonished by the fact that there are pain conditions without any discernible damage at all. We shall discuss two conditions of this kind, both extremely common—headaches and back pain.

HEADACHES

A pain in the head can be classified either as a tension headache or as a migraine. The common tension headache is episodic, and one feels as though muscles are contracting in the front or the back of the head, squeezing the head in a throbbing band. Migraine is felt as a pain on one side of the head; its characteristics are an intense level of pain, nausea, inability to bear light, and an overwhelming need to rest and sleep. Migraine attacks are often preceded by a change of mood and odd sensory and motor changes—one sees flashing or dazzling lights, has difficulty speaking, or cannot move some part of the body. Repeated showers of severe migraine pain are known as cluster headaches.

Most people would say that the cause of a headache is obvious—it is anxiety. Let us pause to consider the use of the word "cause." The question "What is the cause of the light coming from the bulb in the ceiling?" can have two answers, both of which are true. One is that somebody has switched the light on; the other is that an electricity generator is pumping electrons down the line and heating the filament that emits light. Similarly, we can generally identify the worry—or family quarrel, or insoluble problem, or whatever—that has "switched on" a headache. Nevertheless, headaches sometimes appear for no apparent reason, and no amount of heart searching or memory searching can establish a cause of this kind. We have to ask, therefore, what process inside the head makes headaches possible.

In the case of a hangover, we assume that the intake of alcohol produces chemical damage. As a matter of fact, no researcher has ever detected or located this damage, but it may be that we don't yet possess the right technology to do so. Even if the assumption is correct, the alcohol could be the switch for the headache rather than the underlying cause. In the case of headache related to anxiety, no one would suggest that the worry or quarrel has inflicted physical damage on the brain—yet the result is pain.

It has been suggested that the cause of a tension headache is contraction of a muscle, and the experience is in the nature of a muscle cramp. However, investigation shows that muscle contraction (easily detected with electrical recording instruments) occurs after the pain has set in and does not occur extensively enough to explain the pain. Another theory attempted to explain migraine headaches as throbbing in the head in rhythm with the heartbeat (hence, these headaches are sometimes called vascular headaches). But it turned out that changes in the blood vessels, which can be accurately monitored, were out of phase with the pain. We have to conclude, therefore, that these phenomena—muscle contractions and blood vessel changes—are not the *cause* of the pain, but the *result* of a painful process in the head.

What, then, can be the fundamental mechanism whose end-product is a headache? The sensory mechanisms of the body have evolved to an extraordinary level of sensitivity. The ear is so sensitive that it can detect the bombardment of single atoms. The eye is so sensitive that it can detect single photons. The sensory mechanism of the skin can detect and analyze subtle patterns better than any scientific instrument. If we think of our nervous equipment as an alarm system, we recognize that it is incomparably more sensitive than the alarm system you install in your house or your car. Is it any wonder that it sometimes goes off for no reason, or no reason that can be identified? Such a highly sensitive and potentially explosive system can easily be thrown into a temporary pathological state, which lasts until it regains normal stability. Changes in blood pressure and hormonal changes could be the trigger for such an event. Another trigger could be a shift in the endocrine system associated with menstruation or with taking contraceptive pills. Furthermore, migraine has a known genetic component, which itself could be the overdevelopment of excitatory faculties of the sensory system.

All this does not mean that we cannot prevent headaches by dealing with the immediate trigger. It does mean, however, that we have to live with the consequences of possessing an exquisitely sensitive nervous system that occasionally flips its lid. It also means that we have to accept the existence of pain without an external cause in the form of tissue damage.

BACK PAIN

Back pain is such a widespread scourge that, at some point in their lives, more than 60% of employed men and women have been obliged to take time off from work because of it. For most of them, the pain is episodic and disappears after a few days or at most weeks, perhaps to recur after a long interval. But some people—indeed, a considerable number—are never free from back pain. Their lives are ruled, or even wrecked, by the constant pain and by the consequent restriction of movement. The pain feels as though some serious and progressive damage is affecting the back. The worse the pain, and the longer it persists, the more convinced the sufferer becomes of this "obvious" fact, and the more insistent is his demand for remedial action, probably by surgery.

One type of damage that has received much credit (or rather discredit) is the slipped disc (Fig. 5). The disc is the jelly-like substance that cushions the bony surfaces of the vertebrae.

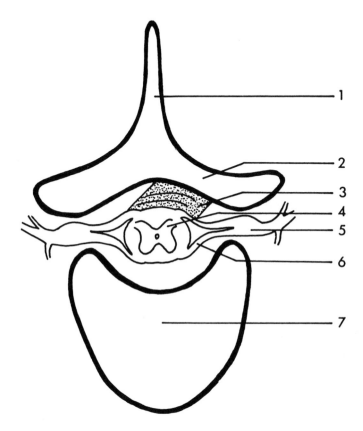

FIGURE 5. A vertebral bone containing the spinal cord. (1) The bony spinous process which points toward the back and can be felt and seen as the row of bumps that run down the midline of the back; (2) the arch of the vertebrum; (3) the epidural space between bone and spinal cord; (4) the spinal cord (see Fig. 4); (5) the dorsal root ganglion that contains the cell bodies of the sensory fibers (3 in Fig. 4); (6) the ventral root that carries the nerve fibers to muscle (9 in Fig. 4); (7) the body of the vertebrum; the disc lies here as a cushion between each body.

It is normally held in place by thick bands of connective tissue. If this tissue becomes weak, the disc bulges out, presses on roots and other substances, and tilts the vertebrae. The result is a combination of pain, numbness, and motor weakness, of the kind we described when discussing nerve damage.

Less well known, but no less troublesome, is spinal stenosis, a condition in which tissue acts to narrow the spinal canal and to compress the roots. This causes pain in the lower back, the buttocks, and the legs. Walking, and even standing, become difficult and intensify the pain, which can be extremely severe, with a burning or vice-like sensation.

Another cause of back pain, which we can describe as tissue damage, is arthritis (erosion) of the joints between the vertebrae. When this occurs, the back is held stiff and often distorted. There is marked stiffness in the morning, somewhat relieved by movement. In addition to the pain in the spine, there may be pain in the buttocks, the thighs, and the feet caused by maintaining the same position.

If we add together these three causes of back pain, and some others that are less common, we can find a credible diagnosis of about 30% of cases of serious back pain. What about the other 70%? In some rich countries, surgeons go ahead and operate without a diagnosis, which may or may not do some good. The puzzle remains: there are many thousands of people, undoubtedly suffering severe pain, in whose bodies no sign of damaged tissue has been detected by the most sophisticated modern diagnostic techniques. The pain can radiate into the groin, the abdomen, the legs, or the perineum, impelling the patient to consult another specialist. It can be so excruciating that standing or even sitting is tolerable only for a few minutes and the sufferer is reduced to lying down all day. How can there be such appalling pain without the possibility of explaining what's wrong? Often, doctors offer the patient an explanation such as a torn muscle or a ripped ligament, although this damage has been deduced rather than actually observed.

It may be that our diagnostic techniques are still not advanced enough to detect all types of damaged tissue. This is quite likely because the existing techniques concentrate on bone and could miss other tissue changes. Even spinal stenosis has been recognized only within the last 25 years. Perhaps some future advance will reveal the presence of the equivalent of a decayed tooth somewhere in the back.

Another possibility is that tissue damage in the past has repaired itself but has left a hyperexcitable area of the nervous system (we have described the long-term effects of nerve damage). This would account for some of the failures of surgery. These failures are unlikely to be the fault of incompetent surgeons, for there is a very low success rate (under 5%) when a failed operation is repeated by a different surgeon. It is more likely that the surgery was carried out too late to prevent the effects of past nerve damage, which set off a cascade of changes in the nervous system.

But the ultimate explanation may be an internal instability in the nervous system. If we can have tension headaches without tissue damage, it is possible to conceive of "tension back pain" without tissue damage. Deep palpation of the muscles of any normal person reveals the presence of particularly tender points. Sometimes, under conditions of stress, anxiety, or sleeplessness, these points become so tender that movement is limited (this is called the myofascial syndrome). A particular version of this condition affects the jaw and neck, although no damaged tissue can be found. The tender points and the muscle contraction are real, but migrate from one area to another. The pain often radiates and is referred to distant areas. It seems that, without any tissue damage, parts of the central and peripheral nervous system have moved to a very high level of excitability. Back pain could be the way in which this excitability finds expression. As the ancient Greek myth teaches us, everyone has an Achilles heel. It could be located in the lower back.

To summarize: the cause of a pain that seems so obvious to

the person who suffers may not be simple. Some serious pains are associated with no apparent damage or injury. Equally, some very obvious injuries and diseases are not associated with pain. We must go on to explain why the nervous system, the brain, and the spinal cord generate this variable link between damage and pain.

3

Childbirth

Pain without Illness

Birth is—matched only by death—the most universal of human experiences. You, the reader, have been involved in it as newborn infant and perhaps as mother; perhaps, also as a witness or helper. Yet this experience has never been and can never be exactly the same for all women and all babies. Each woman, as she approaches childbirth, differs from other women, not only in physical respects, but also in attitude, background, thinking, and expectation. This is the essential fact of human individuality. Another reason for discussing childbirth in some detail is that hardly any aspect of life has gathered such a welter of myths, unproven beliefs, and old wives' tales—myths about pregnancy, about the birth process, and about pain in particular. We need to clear the air by listening to what mothers say.

Medea in Euripides' play says that she would rather stand in line of battle three times than give birth once. Three aspects of her statement are worth comment. She uses the word *poine* for the pains of both battle wounds and childbirth, with the implication that they are ordained, inescapable, and honorable. Second, Medea was a witch, and it is possible that a witch's views on pains and their relative merits might be a little odd.

Finally, Euripides was a man, as are the authors of this book. Can a man write about a pain, a sensory and emotional experience, that he cannot experience? He can accurately report what mothers say, but is that enough? He can try to remove from his report and interpretation those patronizing and patriarchal aspects of his male heritage.

Perhaps one should also ask: "Can a mother write about the pain experienced by other mothers?" The answer is not obvious; each experience is unique, but not so different that it fails to fall into general classes with which one can have understanding and sympathy.

Generally speaking—that is, for the majority of women throughout the world—childbirth is accompanied by a certain amount of pain. This is not surprising. It requires a highly unusual sustained physical effort, placing enormous and quite exceptional strain on the organs, joints, and muscles that are affected. The average woman, unless she is unlucky enough to sustain a serious injury, will never find her body submitted to an equivalent strain for the rest of her life. Hence, no woman should be unduly anxious about the pain that she encounters; still less should she feel guilty about admitting it or imagine that it stamps her as weak or cowardly. At the same time, most women find that the pain is within the limits of the tolerable, some feel no pain at all, and others would say that "pain" is the wrong word for a sensation of purposeful and useful effort. It is already clear that the variations are wide-ranging.

THE PAINS OF PREGNANCY

The birth of a baby is, of course, the culmination of a process that has normally continued for 9 months. It is, indeed, a dual process. One aspect of it is the growth and development of the future baby. Not yet ready for independent life, it is floating in the amniotic fluid within the uterus and is attached by the umbilical cord to the placenta plastered on the inner wall of the womb. The other aspect of the process concerns the mother. Her womb is being steadily enlarged; previously confined entirely within the pelvis, it grows until the top can be felt well above the navel.

The weight of the placenta and amniotic fluid is approximately equal to that of the baby, so that the mother may end up carrying about 16 pounds. This would be the weight of a fair-sized suitcase; given the option, one would not choose to carry a suitcase in front of the belly. The woman finds that she must change her posture to adjust to the unusual burden; adoption of an unaccustomed posture, sustained over a period of time, is inevitably uncomfortable and can even be very painful. Her breathing is less free than it would normally be, because new tissues in her abdomen press up into her chest. Pressure on the pelvis tends to check the flow of blood returning from the legs, and the legs may swell. The new posture may also cause pressure on nerves in this region, resulting in tingling pains and weakness of the legs. Strain on the lower vertebrae of the spine may cause back pain. The sight of a full-term pregnant mother walking with her back overextended to counterbalance her front and with her hand pressed into the small of her back demonstrates the orthopedic postural problems and their painful consequences. To sum up, pain in pregnancy may be the prelude to pain in childbirth. The more there is of one, the more there will probably be of the other.

PREPARATIONS FOR BIRTH

During the final stage of pregnancy, the connective tissue that binds the joints together is loosened by hormonal endocrine changes. The mother is being prepared for the energetic feat that she will soon perform. If she has been having postural problems, she may feel greater discomfort as her joints become more supple. A point on the credit side is that women who normally suffer badly from arthritis may find joyful relief during this time.

The baby, floating freely in the amniotic fluid, will now be kicking or even performing somersaults. This is called quickening, a lovely word that preserves the old use of "quick" to mean "alive" or "lively." (This sense of the word appears in three other phrases: "the quick and the dead," "quicksilver" for mercury, and "the quick of the nails," for the living part.) The baby's head sinks into the pelvis and is held there, stationary, in preparation for birth. This change, known as engagement, makes the mother's situation easier because the top of the womb is lower than it was. In some cases, the baby's bottom settles into the pelvis instead of its head and will emerge first. These breech deliveries are difficult or even hazardous, and when they are in prospect, a cesarean section is usually considered advisable.

The third aspect of preparation for birth is the onset of contractions of the womb—intermittent, fairly weak, but strong in later stages. Although the mother will be aware of these contractions, they are normally painless. The fact that the womb can contract powerfully but without pain gives us an important clue to the origins of the pain that follows in the first stage of labor.

LABOR BEGINS: THE FIRST STAGE

Pressure bursts the membranes; the contractions build up in frequency and intensity; they press directly on the baby's body and force its head into the cervix. Normally closed, the cervix gradually opens to a width of about 4 in. An intravaginal examination can be made to check progress by feeling the extent of cervical dilatation. Slowly, the baby's head advances through the cervix and into the vagina.

It is now that the mother probably experiences the famous "pangs of labor"—episodic pain, associated with the contractions. Centered in the lower abdomen, the pain often spreads in a band encircling the whole body, including the lower back, and radiating down the legs. The baby is also disturbed during the contractions because its blood supply through the placenta is reduced. Between the contractions, the mother may be aware of another kind of pain in her back—steady rather than episodic, and sometimes bad and she certainly feels pain in her lower abdomen.

But here we must pause to ask, "What is the mother doing during this crucial, perhaps exciting, perhaps terrifying period?" The answer depends to an immense extent on the culture in which she lives. In a Western, developed country, she will have entered a hospital. She is expected to be obedient, passive, submissive, and willing to cooperate with the experts in childbirth. She will be told "Take your clothes off and climb onto that bed." Having obeyed, she will lie flat on her back waiting for the next contraction or for whatever else may happen. The scene of this drama is a strange white world dominated by strangers, relieved at best by the presence of a nurse and the (perhaps unfamiliar, perhaps untrustworthy) figure of the obstetrician.

In a different type of culture, such as rural Mexico, the beginning of regular contractions is the signal for the start of a great party. The mother, who of course is at home, is surrounded by singing, dancing, drinking friends and relations. Nobody tells her to lie down and keep still. Whatever she does, and whatever the others do, the baby usually gets born.

Which of these scenes is best for the mother and baby? In the West today, there is much debate on that question but a shortage of hard facts. Obstetricians are beginning to take the common-sense view that what the mother thinks best really is best. If she wants to walk around, why not? If she chooses to stand, to sit, or to curl up alone in a corner, it may well help her and it seems to make little difference to the baby. Indeed, there is growing evidence that lying flat during the contractions increases the steady pain in the back.

THE SECOND STAGE OF LABOR

Now the baby's head emerges from the dilated cervix and begins to advance more rapidly. In doing so, it must displace and stretch some sensitive structures—the vagina, the bladder, and the rectum. It must bulge out the floor of the pelvis and the sensitive skin of the perineum (that is, the region around the anus and vagina). This is a time of crisis and possible danger. One danger is that the placenta's blood supply to the baby via the umbilical cord may be obstructed.

In the second stage, the mother is well aware that a climax is near. The contractions become more violent and sustained. Because the baby is strongly displacing tissue not previously affected, the location of pain shifts to include the pelvis and perineum. Out of this phase of excitement and struggle, the baby is born. The third stage of labor—the expulsion of the placenta—is one of relative relief. The contractions may be quite strong, but the soft placenta passes easily through structures widely dilated by the baby.

THE CAUSES OF PAIN

It is not the uterine contractions themselves which are painful. It is the pressure those contractions exert on sensitive structures, particularly the cervix of the uterus. The nerves that carry signals to the spinal cord run from both sides of the uterus. One group runs along the fallopian tubes over the ovaries while the largest group collect on either side of the cervix (Fig. 6). These nerves end surprisingly high up in the spinal cord in the lower thoracic and upper lumbar segments. That is why mothers in the first stage of labor feel the pains in the small of the back. This is yet another example of referred pain.

As labor progresses, intense pressure begins to be applied to the walls of the vagina itself and to the floor of the pelvis and the vaginal entrance. These structures are supplied by their own sensory nerves, which enter the lowest part of the spinal cord. The main pain now descends and is felt in the structures being distorted.

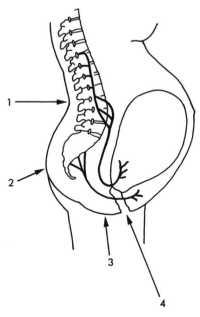

FIGURE 6. Diagram of nerves to the pelvis of a woman approaching delivery. One group of nerves runs from the uterus (womb) to the lower thoracic and upper lumbar vertebrae. A second group runs to the sacral vertebrae. (1) The route and target of needles commonly used to give epidural or spinal anesthetics; (2) the route for caudal block anesthetics; (3 and 4) routes for local anesthesia used for the last stages of labor.

INTRUSIONS AND PAIN

To produce a baby is the personal experience and triumph of the mother. To intrude takes away from the mother some of her pride and some of her sense of control, which is a key factor in her pains. Classical intrusion, the cesarean section, was reserved for the ultimate emergency when the mother was on the point of death and the occasional baby could be "wrenched untimely from the womb." That act produced Julius Caesar and the name of the operation. In the eighteenth century, an extraordinary family of male midwives, the Chamberlains, secretly introduced forceps as a method of manipulating babies out of the womb. They could preserve their family secret from the mothers and other midwives because deliveries of high-class ladies by men were performed discreetly, hidden by skirts and sheets. For two generations, the Chamberlains gained a huge reputation, even wrapping the handles of the forceps in leather so that the clanging of the blades would be silenced. With the technical advances in surgery, anesthesia, and control of infection, the two emergency procedures of cesarean section and high-forceps delivery became standard practice. The emergencies were generally signalled by the recognition that labor was not progressing and that the baby and mother were becoming dangerously distressed.

Now comes the problem. When should intervention occur? Should there be preventive, preemptive intervention? Careful monitoring of the baby while still in the uterus allows earlier and earlier detection of the onset of distress and danger at a stage when no irreversible damage to the baby's brain has occurred. In 1819 René Théophile Laennec invented the stethoscope. Curiously, the motivation was not so much diagnosis as to satisfy the sensibility of rich ladies who objected to having physician's ears pressed to their bodies. Exactly the same social taboo led the Chinese to develop pulse diagnosis, since court women had to be hidden from lower-class physicians. The technological progression from listening intermittently with a stethoscope to continuous electronic fetal heart monitoring is a minor example of the ease of progressive intrusion in the mother. Some mothers like the reassurance that their baby's status is being checked heartbeat by heartbeat. Others resent the depersonalization of wires leading to a shiny box that winks and beeps its interpretation of the baby.

Much more serious is the question of whether (or when) to do a cesarean section. Cautious obstetricians will set more and more sensitive criteria for the onset of difficulties during labor. Further, they begin to predict that there will be trouble and perform the operation before labor starts. This tendency is exaggerated by the fear of litigation. All of this results in a huge, worldwide variation in the rate of cesarean section. It is lowest in poor countries and highest in rich ones, rising to 30% of all deliveries in some parts of the United States.

While the time and place for these major interventions are the subject of debate, in which the mother must participate for her peace of mind, this is equally important for the three common minor interventions. The first of these is artificial induction of labor produced by triggering uterine contraction by injection. With modern diagnostic methods, particularly ultrasound, it is possible to determine exactly when the baby is mature enough to be born safely. However, the precise time when the baby and mother actually decide to launch the baby can be delayed with no great consequence. In addition to considerations of convenience, there are sometimes clear medical reasons for speeding the onset of labor, for example, when partial beginnings produce leaks of amniotic fluid. Babies, of course, carry no wristwatches or appointment diaries, and labor may begin (as it usually does in novels and films) in the middle of the night. The mother may be obliged to go into hospital when she is tired and sleepy, or at an inconvenient time, or when the father is for some reason unable to accompany her. If nurses and doctors change shifts while labor is in progress, the mother is confronted by new faces just when she needs familiar reassurance. For these reasons, some women—especially if they have important jobs or other responsibilities—are likely to welcome induction, which enables them to give birth at a time fixed in advance.

However, when women are urged to accept induction, they are probably right in guessing that one aim is to suit the convenience of the hospital staff, and the mother's wishes are a secondary consideration. Many, probably most, women feel that induction is soulless and mechanical and would be happier to let nature take its course. It should never be forgotten that childbirth is a natural process, not an illness, and there is seldom any justification for hastening it as one would hasten an operation to ward off a threat to health. The golden rule is that the mother should make the choice. If labor is to be induced, it should be only because the mother so decides.

The other two interventions, *low forceps* and *episiotomy*, are largely for relief of the mother's pain and her future comfort. During the last phase of the second stage, the baby becomes freer and freer to advance at surprising speed. In the process, the tissue around the baby's head does not have time to stretch and may tear. In this phase, the mother is encouraged not to push so hard and the baby's head may be held back. Forceps can be fitted gently around the head to ease the twisting, turning final advance. By 1920, this was recommended as a routine in high-class American hospitals. Finally, as the baby's head comes out of the vaginal entrance, a single cut to enlarge the entrance is commonly done. This episiotomy cut is closed by stitches immediately after the birth. In 1918, Pomeroy recommended this cutting and reconstructing of the perineum in every primipara (first birth) in order to reduce compression of the baby's head and for the mother's comfort. By 1980, a British survey showed 65% of mothers have episiotomies. The reason given by the doctors for this common practice is safer delivery and less pain after birth. Unfortunately, as with so much common and common-sense practice, there is no evidence of these effects.

We have presented the details of labor not as an obstetric textbook, but because a mother's ease depends on understanding and the sense of control it brings. The pains of her labor help no one, certainly not the baby. Her freedom to play her part in delivery and nursing requires that she is not dominated by pain.

WHAT MOTHERS SAY

So much for the physical processes of childbirth. These processes vary in each individual case for a number of reasons, such as the size and build of the mother, whether she has given birth before, and the size of the baby. Beyond that, women speak of their sensory and emotional experiences with a certain common comradeship, but with marked differences. How are we to describe what mothers have in common, their individual differences, and the reasons for these differences?

On this subject, every mother can speak with an authority based on her own experiences. She may even insist that she is speaking not only of what she felt, but of what all other women ought to feel. Men have listened to these grand generalizations and, as is their wont, have added their own authoritarian statements about proper behavior. A woman expecting her first baby is inevitably subjected to education regarding what is normal and what is correct. Depending on whom she listens to, she will anticipate that there will be terrible pain, or that the pain will be controllable and tolerable, or that (if she follows the right advice) she can escape pain altogether. But what actually happens?

Earlier, we explained the McGill Pain Questionnaire, which evaluates pain according to the words used by the sufferer to describe it (41). The sensory words most often used to describe pain in childbirth are *sharp, cramping, aching, throbbing, stabbing, hot, shooting, tight, heavy*. With regard to emotional affect, 49% of women answering the questionnaire used the word *tiring* and 36% used the word *exhausting*.

Women giving birth for the first time (known as primiparas) experience more pain than women who have had other children (multiparas). On the McGill scale, the average primipara suffered pain rated at 35 and the average multipara at 30. For comparison, people with broken bones average scores of 20 and cancer patients, 27. Scores above 35 were recorded only in cases of nerve injuries and traumatic amputation, which are recognized as extremely painful conditions. So the evidence is that the pain of childbirth ranks high in the range of human experience.

We must remember, however, that these averages conceal

wide individual variations. Indeed, the individual variation for childbirth pain is much greater than in other situations, such as pain in cancer. Of primiparas in Canada, 9.2% described their pain as mild, 29.5% as moderate, 37.9% as severe, and 23.4% as excruciating. A study of Scandinavian women (despite their reputation for toughness and stoicism) yielded a similar result.

As we have seen, a normal birth is a predictable, well-ordered progression from stage to stage. It seems logical to assume that the pain follows a steadily rising curve throughout the process. As a (male) poet wrote: "When the pain is sorest the child is born." There is some truth in this picture; primiparas in the Canadian sample, on the average, rated their pain at 20 some 12 hours before birth and 40 just before delivery. But again, these are averages. Some women experience their worst pains early in the process; some describe the pain in terms of surprising, irregular peaks and troughs.

The intermittent character of childbirth pain is stressed in the evocative account to be found in Doris Lessing's novel *A Proper Marriage*. The writer is describing the hospital experience of her heroine, Martha Quest, a healthy young primipara:

> The stars vanished in another hot wave of pain. . . . She felt the baby knot and propel itself down; it recoiled and slacked, and she with it. The pain had changed. She could mark the point at which, just as it abruptly changed its quality a couple of hours before in the bath, so now it ground into a new gear, as it were. It gripped first her back, then her stomach, then it was as if she and the baby were being wrung out together by a pair of enormous steel hands. . . . The watch that lay six inches from her nose on her crooked arm said that the pains were punctual at two minutes. But from the moment that the warning hot wave of pain swept up her back, she entered a place where there was no time at all. An agony so unbelievable gripped her that her astounded and protesting mind cried out that it was impossible such pain could be. It was a pain so violent that it was no longer pain, but a condition of being. Every particle of flesh shrieked out, while the wave spurted like an electric current from somewhere in her backbone and went through her in shock after shock. The wave

receded, however, just as she had decided she would disinte-
grate under it. . . . She went limp into a state of perfect painlessness, an exquisite exhaustion in which the mere idea of pain
seemed impossible—it was impossible that it could recur again.
And as soon as the slow flush of sensation began, the condition
of painlessness seemed as impossible as the pain had seemed
only a few moments before. They were two states of being,
utterly disconnected, without a bridge.

Directly after the birth of a child, there is no pain. The co-
author (P.W.) remembers hearing a hardened and cynical male
obstetrician say, "All women look like angels at this moment." It
is true. The woman whose face a short while before was
distorted and sweating, who was uttering curses or prayers, is
transformed into serenity, relief, and triumph. She falls into a
sleep of satisfied exhaustion. But the next day is different again.
She feels new pains, the consequence of the effort and struggle
from which she has to recover.

It is interesting at this point to ask her to describe her
experience, and even more interesting to eavesdrop on her
conversation with her first visitors, especially her own mother.
Many women give very precise accounts of their labor, which
tally well with what they said at the time. With some, however,
this is the time for mythmaking. One woman gave her mother a
graphic account, contraction by contraction, of how she endured mounting agony but in the end triumphantly gave birth
in spite of being completely ignored by the unfeeling midwives
and doctors; in fact, she had been deeply anesthetized throughout her delivery. A sort of maternal counterpart to male ma-
chismo sometimes generates phrases like "Nothing to it," "A
piece of cake," or "You just squeeze a few times and out pops
the baby." Mythical accounts and realistic reports compete with
each other to produce family histories—and to shape the expec-
tations of the mothers of the next generation.

Myths are not innocent expressions of childhood fantasy;
rather, they codify beliefs that provide the mythmaker with an
identity. They distinguish *us* from *them*, using pain and suffer-

ing as markers. *We* are tough, brave, rational people who think and live properly. *They* are cowardly, irresponsible people who do all the wrong things from a combination of ignorance and stupidity. Therefore, *we* do not suffer pain; *they* do.

WHO SUFFERS?

Which women do, in reality, suffer more pain in childbirth than other women? First, as we have noted, primaparas experience more pain than multiparas. Second, poor women report worse pain than rich women. There may be several reasons for this (aside from the fact that rich women get better analgesia, but this factor was excluded in the relevant studies). The poorer women may have had a history of ill health, may have had inferior medical care, and may have strained their joints and muscles by arduous work in the home or in the factory. Another reason is that rich women tend to start a family later than poor women; a research finding that may surprise some readers is that older mothers report less pain than younger ones. Surprisingly too—and disappointingly—women seem to experience more pain when the baby's father is present in the delivery room than when he is not. Possibly, pain is made more acute by unconscious resentment at the sight of the pain-free male who is responsible for the pregnancy. Perhaps there is something to be said for the traditional custom of *couvade*, whereby the man wills himself into sharing the woman's pain.

Women with a history of painful and disturbing menstrual periods are more likely to suffer pain in childbirth, although the two processes are quite different. Some people, particularly men, will dismiss the women concerned as helpless individuals who complain about everything, but others will reflect more seriously on an observation for which there is no obvious reason. In any event, the link between vulnerability to one kind of pain and vulnerability to another kind gives us a significant clue to the causes of individual variation.

A "fact" widely believed in developed nations is that most women in primitive societies—or in the Third World as we say today—give birth painlessly. We enclose the word "fact" in quotation marks because this notion is quite devoid of truth. It can be traced to the general belief, dominant for centuries, that "primitive" or "savage" races lacked the sensibilities of the "higher" white races. Clearly, this was a very convenient belief for colonial officials and plantation owners, since it meant that the people in question didn't "feel as we do" when they toiled all day in the hot sun, sweated under heavy loads, or were flogged for offenses against the rules. Many tales were told of women working in the fields, who stepped into the bushes, gave birth, and resumed work. Seldom was it remembered that they may have had no option, nor was it remembered that a certain proportion of multiparas in any society gave birth very rapidly (as ambulance drivers can tell you). Sadly, some of the undernourished women who stepped into the bushes may have been giving birth to small, premature babies—the sort of babies who die easily. And some may have been giving birth through a cervix still torn during another unattended delivery the year before. Poor people everywhere are inadequately prepared for childbirth and receive little or no aftercare for tearing or infection. Let us add that these mothers generally did not speak the language of the ruling classes, and there are few records of what they experienced or felt.

The idea that black or brown people are impervious to pain because they are innately different is a crude form of racism that is now, let us hope, thoroughly discredited. But the belief lingers on in another form, stemming perhaps from eighteenth-century visions of idyllic "happy islands" where life was simple, relaxed, and uncomplicated. In the absence of the tensions and conflicts of modern society, we are sometimes told, anxieties are reduced and childbirth, consequently, is painless.

Professor J. J. Bonica, a pioneer in the study of pain, has demonstrated conclusively that ethnic origin has nothing to do with liability to childbirth pain (8). In a Seattle hospital, women of Asian origin—even including Vietnamese who had recently arrived in the United States—experienced pain in childbirth and requested analgesia just as often as other women. In a survey made in New England hospitals, detailed studies of black and white mothers failed to reveal any difference along ethnic lines.

When differences are observed, it generally turns out on closer inquiry that these are differences in behavior, or simply in communication, not in the actual experience. Turkana women on the Kenya–Sudan border behaved calmly during birth and demonstrated no pain; however, in reply to questions they said that the process had been very painful, but they would have lost social face if they had shown it. Mojave (North American Indian) women had experienced a great deal of pain and had avoided showing what they felt out of fear of ridicule. At the other extreme, Bonica visited a large maternity hospital in Turin in 1954 and found that "the labour ward was a scene of cacaphony caused by the screaming, pleading and praying of nearly fifty laboring women." But, on a return visit 5 years later, he heard only an occasional moan; this time, the women had been through an intensive course of psychoprophylaxis (mental preparation). All the same, most of them said afterward that they had suffered moderate or severe pain.

The simple fact, often overlooked or distorted by myth and fantasy, is that pain is a private experience but reaction to pain is culturally determined. What you say about pain to other people depends on who you are—and on who they are. Proper behavior is decided by the society, community, or family, not by the individual. Eleanor Roosevelt wrote, "I was brought up in the sort of family where one did not have a headache when guests were expected." But in a different kind of family, anyone suffering pain or injury was expected to shout loudly to attract attention. A lonely woman in an alien culture, unable to speak the language or make the accepted signals, is in real trouble. Desperation may cause her to scream in terror or to huddle up in silent misery. If no differences were observed between black and white mothers in a New England hospital, this does not mean that they came from the same culture. It means that they all entered a new common culture—the dominating culture of the hospital, which, in a few days, wipes out their cultural heritage.

However, generalizations about culture are a favorite sport with both the scientific and the literary fraternity. Jews are this, Italians are that, and Russians are something else. In reality, such differences as exist are largely in styles of expression or behavior. The interaction of ethnic background and the expression of pain has been particularly well studied in the United States (21, 63). For example, a group of young women born in the United States volunteered to rate electric shocks as only just detectable, painful, or as strong as they were willing to tolerate. Their families were Irish, Italian, Jewish, or "Yankee" in origin, and they differed in the degree of shock they were willing to tolerate and in how they coped. Furthermore, they changed their criteria when challenged with a reminder of their ethnic origin. When black, Irish, Italian, Jewish, and "WASP" women were questioned about the intensity of pain in childbirth, no difference was detected. However, in a study of 536 cancer patients with European origins, the same level of pain was reported regardless of ethnic origin, but the affective response was less in patients of English, German, and Scandinavian origin. The amount of pain seems common to all of us, but our culture is one of the influences that affect our methods of coping and of expression.

"NATURAL CHILDBIRTH"

Five decades ago, Dr. Grantly Dick Read launched the movement for "natural childbirth" or "childbirth without fear" (17). The ideas that he advanced, since taken up and extended by many others, were both revolutionary and constructive—but, like all of us, Dick Read was a child of his times. He wrote:

"Among less cultured races, I saw painless effort and happiness combined in childbirth. I saw a woman walk away from a harvest field, exalted and laughing, with her baby wrapped in a cloth: her baby less than half an hour old." The "savages" or "pagans" had become "less cultured races," but the picture was similar.

Dick Read was led by such observations, and by his considerable experience as an obstetrician, to ask four questions: "Why is labor so frequently painful? Why is interference so often resorted to? Why are so many drugs used? Why should a woman be mentally dulled or unconscious of the arrival of her child?" He concluded: "The art of conducting physiological labor depends on the attendant's ability to break down and prevent the occurrence of the vicious circle of fear, pain and tension." When a child is being born, he pointed out, there are three labors—physical on the mother's part, emotional on the mother's part, and physical on the attendant's part.

As seen by Dick Read, childbirth is a painless, joyful experience, provided the mother is properly prepared for it. If a normal childbirth is not painless, either the attendant (doctor or nurse) has failed or else the mother has failed to pay attention to the attendant. These are simple, definite, powerful statements. No one would question that it is good to combat fear and ignorance. There is, indeed, ample evidence that pain is intensified by feelings of fear or anxiety. But, like Dick Read in his day, we have a duty to doubt, question, and test the accepted wisdom—including the concept of painless natural childbirth.

The best way to do this is to hear the evidence of mothers: both those who are untrained and those who have received instruction and training in obstetric physiology, breathing exercises, and relaxation techniques. There is no doubt that each of these aspects of training is a good idea, in that they reduce fear, teach the usefulness of distraction, and improve physical fitness. The only issue we wish to discuss here is their effect on the amount of pain that the mother experiences. Professor Ronald Melzack carried out such a study in Montreal and found that women who chose to have childbirth training recorded significantly lower pain scores than those who did not (41). So far, so good—but the average scores of both groups were still regrettably high (33 on the McGill scale for the trained mothers, 37 for the untrained). Some instructors were more effective than others, but the prize winner produced an average score of only 26 in his group, comparable to the pain scores of cancer sufferers. In untrained and in trained groups, the same proportion of women asked for an epidural anesthetic during labor. Multiparas experienced less pain than primaparas, but this was true in both untrained and trained groups.

After the struggle was over, and after the admission of pain, the trained mothers tended to feel guilty. They felt that they had let themselves down, they had let their teachers down, and they had failed by requesting drugs that might perhaps be damaging to their babies. Had they, however, really failed? Or had they been misled by a novel doctrine that declared too dogmatically that childbirth should be painless?

There is not a shadow of doubt that preparation for childbirth is effective and beneficial. It has produced two revolutionary changes in the attitudes of mothers and of those who have the task of helping them. First, since childbirth is more than simply "doing what comes naturally," a mother needs knowledge, understanding, and assistance. Second, she needs—and deserves—a sense of control; she is a key member of her own delivery team. But this outlook ought not to require her to believe that if she experiences pain, it is the result of her failure to overcome her fears, or that women in simpler societies enjoy freedom from pain. The woman in childbirth—like other people confronting pain—should prepare herself to understand and to cope; she should also recognize herself as an individual with no obligation to conform to an externally imposed norm.

RELIEF OF THE PAINS

It must be added that she needs, and has a right to, relief from pain when it becomes intolerable. Queen Victoria—

mother of nine children, arbiter of right and wrong in the age that bears her name, and a woman who could never be accused of weakness—decided that chloroform was preferable to excessive pain in childbirth. As a matter of fact, unlimited use of chloroform in the nineteenth-century manner was dangerous to mother and child, so the Queen was lucky to suffer no ill effects. Since her time, careful research has led to the development of methods of controlling pain without endangering life.

With extraordinary foresight, James Simpson, who had introduced the anesthesia used by Queen Victoria, wrote in 1848, "If we could induce local anesthesia without the temporary absence of consciousness which is found in the state of general anesthesia, many would regard it as a still greater improvement." It was not until 1884 that Carl Koller and Sigmund Freud discovered the local anesthetic properties of cocaine, and only in 1901 was the first spinal local anesthetic during labor given by Kreis.

The simplest technique for controlling pain is very light anesthesia under the mother's control. She is given a mask and a small compressed-gas cylinder containing a mixture of nitrous oxide and oxygen. When she presses the mask onto her face and breathes deeply, she does not lose consciousness but gains a level of analgesia (relief from pain) that blunts the intensity of a wave of pain. It is impossible for her to overdose herself or to harm her baby, and even if she falls asleep, the mask slips off. Women tend to use it at the peak of a contraction. The fact that the mother controls the analgesic and thus participates in the labor process considerably raises her morale.

If the pain increases in severity and the mother asks for help, she may be given a narcotic by injection. The most favored narcotic has the generic name of pethidine and is known in the United States as Demerol. Probably, rather than having a direct effect on pain, it induces drowsiness and thus makes the sensation of pain less acute. This procedure carries risks, of which doctors are well aware. The drug can depress respiration, and this affects the baby as well as the mother. The baby's first act on being cut off from the mother's blood supply is to start breathing; if it fails to do so, it will die of asphyxia. (This is why babies are more or less blue at birth; they turn pink when they breathe and cry.) If the drug has reduced the baby's ability to breathe, the action of the drug can be instantly neutralized by another drug. Narcotics make childbirth pains much more bearable and have a wonderful effect on afterpains. Also, a narcotic injection can be useful in an unexpected way: by preventing the mother from breathing too violently, it can keep the proportions of oxygen and carbon dioxide in her blood, and therefore in the blood she supplies to the baby until birth, at a normal level.

As can be seen, it is all a matter of judgment. One effect of a narcotic injection is to make thinking processes less clear and cloud the memory, so that the mother emerges with a rather hazy recollection of events.

Local anesthesia has become a more and more common practice for pain control in labor. Local anesthetic agents block the passage of pain-producing impulses on their way to the spinal cord, just as dentists block nerves from the teeth. As we have said, the relevant nerves change as labor progresses. In the early stages, the pain-producing impulses originate from the uterus and cervix. They flow in nerves that leave the side of the uterus and enter the spinal cord in the upper lumbar and lower thoracic area (Fig. 6). They can be blocked by injection on either side of the cervix (paracervical). A more convenient and more frequently employed method is to block them as they enter the spinal cord (lumbar epidural in Fig. 6). A needle or catheter is placed in the space between the bone of the vertebrae and the spinal cord (Fig. 5). Satisfactory relief of pain is achieved, while the mother remains fully aware and the baby is unaffected. The side effects are few. With older methods the block also affected the motor nerves, so that there was some temporary leg weakness and the mother therefore had less control over the pushing activity.

Unfortunately, this almost ideal form of pain relief is not

available to all mothers. In Britain, for example, because of the shortage of trained anesthesiologists, 50% of mothers find that they cannot be offered an epidural block. As is so often the case, the best that medicine has to offer is restricted to the leading hospitals in the most prosperous countries. Britain is highly unlikely to double its tally of anesthesiologists in the near future. To give all mothers adequate relief from pain, we shall need not only scientific research into new methods, but also social changes, so that the safe and simple methods are available without the necessity for highly trained specialists.

As the baby advances through the cervix, new nerves become the major signal carriers. These end in the sacral (lower) spinal cord. The impulses can be blocked by injection around the pudendal nerve (Fig. 6) or as they enter the spinal cord (caudal in Fig. 6) by epidural anesthesia. These techniques allow the site of analgesia to descend as the baby descends, so that pain relief keeps pace. This relief is a blessing for the mother, who can genuinely participate in her own achievement. Moreover, while it has no effect on the strength of the uterine contractions, it greatly reduces the burden on her heart and lungs. If the baby is at risk because of other mishaps, this normalization is particularly important. And if an emergency makes a cesarean section necessary, mother and baby are in much better shape to withstand the ordeal.

Still, the fact remains that an epidural block is a radical medical intervention. The mother has a right and a duty to make an informed decision as to whether she desires such an intervention. Even when all the options are available, she is not truly free to choose unless she understands all the factors involved and the good and bad aspects of each technique. She has a right to intelligent explanation, not to dictation by authoritarian fanatics or even by well-meaning fools. We stress again our major theme: the relief of pain depends to a great extent on an understanding of the nature and cause of pain, because understanding leads to participation and a sense of control.

4

Paradoxes of Pain

During the Crimean War (1854–1856), a young Russian officer, Count Leo Tolstoy, was on duty in the besieged town of Sevastopol. He had already begun his literary career and, with a view to writing a book about the war, made careful notes of everything he observed. One day, he visited the emergency hospital in the Sevastopol Assembly Hall. In his book *Sevastopol Sketches*, Tolstoy records this conversation:

> "Where are you wounded?" you inquire hesitantly and timidly of a gaunt old soldier. . . .
> "In the leg," he answers; but you notice from the folds of his blanket that one of his legs has been amputated up to the thigh. "I'm all right now, thank God," he adds. "I'm waiting for my discharge."
> "Were you wounded long ago?"
> "Nigh on six weeks ago, your honor."
> "Well, does it hurt now?"
> "No, it doesn't hurt any more. It's all right. Only, I feel as if my calf aches when the weather's bad; otherwise it's all right."
> "How did you come to be wounded?"
> "It was in Bastion Five, your honor, during the first bombardment. I had trained my gun and was just going to the next embrasure, when he hit me in the leg. I felt as if I had tumbled down a hole. I looked and found my leg was gone."
> "Didn't you feel any pain at the first moment?"

"No, I didn't. I only felt as if something hot had whipped my leg."

"Well, and afterwards?"

"It wasn't so bad afterwards, either, except when they started pulling the skin over. It was pretty bad then. The main thing's *not to think a lot*, your honor. When you don't think, it's all right. Most trouble comes because a man thinks."

Later in the nineteenth century, the French novelist Emile Zola made notes on conversations with railwaymen. His novel *La Bête Humaine* had a railwayman as its central character and included many details from the railway life. In it, he described a rail crash and the ensuing rescue work:

> The work called for the utmost caution. . . . There were injured whose head and shoulders only protruded from the mass. They were caught as is in a vice, howling with pain. It took a quarter of an hour to get out one man, who made no complaint, but was white as a sheet, assuring them he was all right, not hurt at all, but in fact was minus his legs, and died at once, suffering from such shock that he did not even observe his own horrible mutilation. From a third-class coach which had caught fire they extracted a whole family. The father's and mother's knees were injured, the grandmother had a broken arm, but none of them felt their hurt. They were sobbing and crying for their little girl, fair-haired they said, just turned three, who had vanished under the wreckage.

In both of these passages, we have accounts of people who suffered severe—even, in one case, lethal—injury, of a kind that one would normally expect to be extremely painful, but who felt no pain. Indeed, it is possible to collect quite a number of such accounts, some by writers such as Tolstoy and Zola, some by medical researchers who have investigated the phenomenon of injury without pain. Not surprisingly, accounts by the people who actually experienced the injury are rarer, but we will cite four.

1. On March 30, 1981, President Ronald Reagan survived an assassination attempt when a high-velocity bullet, fired at

short range, entered his chest. At first, it was not clear that the bullet had hit the President at all. He showed signs of faintness, but these were attributed to the sharp impact when Secret Service agents hustled him into his car. Talking later to the press, the President remarked: "A gunshot wound doesn't always give an immediate sense of pain. I've only had one before in the movies, and there you always react as if you were hurt immediately." (Of course, Reagan was not really injured on the movie lot, but as a good actor he simulated the assumed pain.)

2. A London Transport policeman, Steve Hanson, had both arms badly burned while rescuing people from a fire at King's Cross underground rail station in 1987. Interviewed for television in hospital, he said, "No, I didn't feel any pain at the time."

3. One of the co-authors (P.D.W.) was struck on the forehead by a stone while watching a political demonstration in 1976 that led to a clash between demonstrators and police. The stone made a bad gash, which bled profusely and later required stitches. He felt no pain either at the time of the injury or when taken to hospital, but a dull headache set in when it occurred to him that there might be further problems, such as infection. By next morning, he was feeling pain to a distressing degree. It died down as the wound healed cleanly, but he found himself unusually listless, sleepy, irritable, unable to concentrate, and uninterested in food or company. These aftereffects lasted for about 10 days.

4. A classic account of injury without pain comes from Dr. David Livingstone, the famous missionary and explorer. While traveling in Africa, he met a lion and shot it twice, but it nevertheless sprang at him. In his book *Missionary Travels*, Livingstone wrote:

> He caught my shoulder as he sprang, and we both came to the ground together. Growling horribly close to my ear, he shook me as a terrier dog does a rat. The shock produced a stupor

similar to that which seems to be felt by a mouse after the first shake of the cat. It caused a sort of dreaminess, in which there was no sense of pain nor feeling of terror, though quite conscious of all that was happening. It was like what patients partially under the influence of chloroform describe, who see all the operation but feel not the knife.

Luckily for Livingstone (and for his readers), it was the lion that collapsed and died, having been mortally wounded by the bullets fired a minute before. It seems possible that the lion too had experienced injury without immediate pain. As for Livingstone, his injuries were real and serious. He recorded: "Besides crunching the bone into splinters, he left eleven teeth wounds on the upper part of my arm."

In fact, there is no necessary connection between the seriousness of an injury and the feeling of pain. In the sixteenth century, the French essayist Michel de Montaigne wrote, "We are more sensible of one little touch of the surgeon's lancet than of twenty wounds with the sword in the heat of the fight." In modern wars, doctors have noted that wounded soldiers complain of the painful jab when given an injection. A curious case was that of a man who felt no pain when he lost a foot in an industrial accident, but complained of a painful cramp in the *other* leg while he was waiting to be operated on.

The paradoxical phenomenon of injury without pain has been the subject of a number of studies. One was made in World War II by Dr. Henry K. Beecher, who later became the first Professor of Anesthetics at Harvard (incidentally, he was a descendant of Harriet Beecher Stowe). As a colonel in charge of admissions at an Army hospital, he made observations on American soldiers who had been badly wounded in the fighting on the Anzio beachhead. He was astonished to find that only one man in three felt enough pain to require morphine on arrival at the field hospital. The others either said that they were in no pain, or that the pain was quite tolerable without medication.

In 1982, the co-author (P.D.W.) and two colleagues made a study of 138 people who received treatment in the emergency clinic of a large hospital in Montreal (43). The patients included men and women between the ages of 16 and 85; the injuries were varied and resulted from work accidents, home accidents, road accidents, falls on icy street surfaces, or fights. Fifty-one of the patients (37%) said that they felt no pain at the moment of injury. There was some correlation between the seriousness of the injury and the pain (in that 53% of the superficial injuries, but only 28% of the deep-tissue injuries, were pain-free), but this correlation did not hold true in every case. Pain was experienced at various times after the injury—sometimes only a few minutes, generally about an hour, in some cases up to 9 hours. In the case of a man with a broken nose, the time-lapse was over 5 hours. One unexpected finding was that most of the patients described their pain by using words classified as "sensory" in the McGill Pain Questionnaire and few used "affective" words which would indicate an emotional reaction.

CONGENITAL ANALGESIA

It is worth noting at this point that some people are absolutely incapable of feeling pain. This condition is called congenital analgesia. One such individual, known in medical literature as Miss C., was the subject of thorough observation because her father was a Canadian doctor. As a child, she was burned when she climbed onto a hot radiator to look out the window; the scars of burning remained on her legs, but she felt no pain. She also bit off the tip of her tongue, quite painlessly. Another recorded case concerns a little girl who broke her arm at the age of 3, broke her nose at the same age, broke it again at the age of 5, and severely burned her buttocks on an electric heater at the age of 7—all without any pain. This series of accidents would be phenomenal for an ordinary child, but then, an ordinary child would be more careful.

When Miss C. became a student, her father informed the university of her peculiarity and she volunteered to undergo various tests. She was given electric shocks and immersed in an ice bath; never did she show any signs of pain. In one test, a hot lightspot was beamed onto her arm. A normal person would flinch and pull the arm away. Miss C. said, "This is getting pretty hot, and if I don't take my arm away I'll get a burn." Lacking an automatic reaction, she had substituted deliberate thought.

One might be tempted to think of congenital analgesia as the gift of a good fairy. Analgesic children can easily be winners in boisterous games or playground battles, and one of them became a trampoline champion. Sad to say, however, congenital analgesia is more like a witch's curse. Normal people protect or rest a damaged joint after an injury, for instance, by limping in reaction to an ankle sprain. A person who feels no pain and is therefore unaware of the injury goes on using the limb. This causes a breakdown of the joint surface and a consequent risk of infection. Dead or dying tissue is the perfect culture medium for bacteria and is the most likely place for infection to develop. Because blood flow is impaired, the tissue is isolated from the body's defense mechanisms. The infection is then free to extend into nearby bone structures, producing osteomyelitis, which is difficult to treat, because even powerful antibiotics cannot penetrate from the bloodstream. Miss C. developed osteomyelitis and died at the age of 29.

Congenital analgesia presents a challenge to the thinking of physicians and psychologists and its causes are not yet understood (59). It demonstrates in the most dramatic way possible that pain does not automatically follow from injury. It does not, however, explain the frequent occurrence of injury without pain. It would be absurd to suppose that the majority of the soldiers wounded at Anzio, or 37% of the casualties at the Montreal hospital, had congenital analgesia, which is actually very rare. A person with this condition never feels pain, no matter how much time may pass after the injury. The normal person may feel no *immediate* pain, but does feel pain (as the Montreal study showed) after a certain lapse of time.

EXPLAINING THE PARADOX

Various explanations have been suggested for the absence of immediate pain. Each makes sense in some cases, but none is valid in every possible case. The most obvious explanation is that a badly injured person goes into a state of shock, or trauma (both Zola and Dr. Livingstone use the word "shock" in their accounts). But many people have been observed talking calmly and rationally after an injury, and showing none of the recognized signs of shock (such as sweating or shivering)—and yet feeling no pain.

Dr. Beecher considered that the soldiers at Anzio felt no pain because their reaction to being wounded was one of relief (6). A wounded soldier is thankful not to have been killed; he will be carried away from the scene of danger by the stretcher bearers, he can expect a period of rest and care in hospital, and perhaps he will be out of the war for good. The relief may be so great as to leave no room for pain. A few hours later, when safety is taken for granted, pain does set in. Beecher's opinion was strengthened when he returned to his civilian practice and found that the numbers of the pain-free injured were much smaller (of patients undergoing surgery and suffering tissue damage comparable to that of the wounded soldiers, 80% were in severe pain and asked for morphine).

The relief theory sounds convincing, but cannot be wholly satisfactory. Many of the patients at the Montreal hospital were depressed by their experiences, or expressed regret for their careless or foolish behavior, or spoke of unpleasant consequences of the accident, such as time off work and loss of wages or the destruction of a valuable car. Not surprisingly, none of them expressed any pleasure at the accident.

A quite different—indeed, diametrically opposed—theory is that severe injury induces a sense of hopelessness. Dr. Livingstone thought that he was sure to be killed by the lion, and later, reflecting on the state of painlessness and "dreaminess" when he believed he was about to die, he wrote, "This peculiar state is probably produced in all animals killed by the carnivora." Being a devout Christian, he added, "If so, it is a merciful provision by our benevolent Creator for lessening the pain of death." Whether or not we subscribe to Livingstone's theology, his observation has a ring of truth. If we watch a film of a zebra being killed by a lion, there does appear to be more helpless resignation and less frantic struggling on the zebra's part than we might expect. But of course, there is no reason for hopelessness when we sustain a relatively minor injury, like most people in the Montreal study.

One good reason for painlessness at the moment of injury could be absorption in a purpose that demands total concentration. Any doctor or nurse can give examples of people who injured themselves while repairing tiles on a roof or cutting metal with a lathe, but did not feel or even observe the injury until the task was completed. A soldier in battle may be unaware of a wound until the enemy position is captured. A sportsman or athlete may fail to notice a muscle strain until the time comes for relaxation.

A good true story illustrates the point. A champion racehorse called Henbit, competing in the Epsom Derby in 1980, stumbled and broke a bone in the right forefoot when 300 yards from the winning post. Henbit's reaction was to race away and win the Derby, recording the second fastest time in 40 years. Once the race was over, Henbit was seen to be agitated, limping, and evidently in pain. Despite being given the best of veterinary attention, this remarkable horse competed in only one other race, and came in last. We can also observe that a deer that has been shot and wounded by a hunter dashes away at a high speed, exactly like a deer that has been alarmed but not hit. But if you were to find the wounded deer deep in the forest a day later, you would find it apathetic and incapable of movement.

Related to the sense of purpose is the sense of concern for others. Zola wrote of the parents and grandmother who did not feel their injuries because "they were sobbing and crying for their little girl." At the scene of a fire or an earthquake, injured rescue workers are often unaware of pain so long as they are desperately engaged in trying to help the helpless. It can be said with considerable truth that pain at the moment of injury is an indication of an enclosed situation—that is, a situation that is not part of a sequence and involves no one but the injured person. If you fall downstairs and hit your head, there is no reason why you should not feel immediate pain. (Nevertheless, some people in Montreal who slipped on the ice and bruised themselves *did not* feel immediate pain, for whatever reason.)

The best generalization we can make is that human beings—and animals too—behave in the way that is appropriate and useful in given circumstances. If it is desirable, or indeed necessary, to escape from danger, to complete a task, or to assist other people, then this objective would be defeated were we to allow consciousness to be dominated by pain. On the other hand, if the appropriate behavior is to seek rest with a view of recovery, pain is permissible and natural.

PHANTOM LIMB PAIN

While observers such as Tolstoy and Zola noticed that pain was not always a direct consequence of injury, the causative connection was accepted as an axiom by medical authorities well into the twentieth century. We have already quoted a distinguished professor at The Johns Hopkins University who defines pain as "that sensory experience evoked by stimuli that injure or threaten to destroy tissue." Yet there are many examples of pain being experienced without anything that could be called a stimulus. One of these is the phenomenon known as phantom limb pain.

The eloquent phrase "phantom limb" was coined by Weir Mitchell, a U.S. Army physician who had served with the Union forces in the Civil War (47). After amputations, he observed that the man who had lost an arm or leg continued to feel pain, not only in the remaining stump but, it seemed, in an invisible limb that hovered where the lost limb used to be. We recall the words of Tolstoy's soldier: "I feel as if my calf aches when the weather's bad." Admiral Nelson mentioned, in a letter to a friend, that he could still feel the arm he had lost in the battle of Tenerife; he took this as evidence for the eternity of his soul. (The amputation, probably unnecessary, had been clumsily performed in confusion and darkness; the pain must have been atrocious.) But the earliest reference to phantom limb pain comes from the pen of Ambroise Paré (1510–1590), a notable French army surgeon. He wrote in one of his books (we quote from the translation made in 1665):

> Verily it is a thing wondrous strange and prodigious, which will scarcely be credited, unless by such as have seen with their eyes and heard with their ears the patients who have many months after the cutting away of the leg grievously complained that they yet felt exceeding great pain of that leg so cut off.

If a limb is lost for whatever reason—warfare, accident, or surgery—the victim always experiences a feeling that the missing limb is still there. The word "phantom" may give the impression that the amputee is speaking of some vague, misty illusion. In fact, the feeling of reality is so strong that some amputees step out with a missing leg in an unthinking moment. Even the fitting of an artificial limb or prosthesis does not abolish this feeling. Many report such sensations as pins and needles, prickling, constant electric current, contractions, itchiness, or pressure. It is not necessary to lose a limb to have this phantom sensation. If the arm is anesthetized by infiltrating all the nerves at the top of the arm with a local anesthetic, the patient has a very real and astonishing sense of possessing a new arm, even though he can see the old arm (10).

An even more bizarre effect is that the phantom limb takes up strange, impossible positions. This phenomenon has been the subject of a special study. However, most of us have experienced a sensation that can at least be called curious. When you go to the dentist and he injects a local anesthetic, the lip feels numb. On leaving the dentist, you quickly realize that this numb lip makes a claim on your attention. It feels swollen, so you keep poking it with your finger or peering at it in a mirror. That is a phantom lip. The brain has reacted to the absence of the normal nerve signals from the lip and rings gentle alarm signals, telling you that all is not well and you should investigate.

To feel something that does not exist is disturbing. To tell an old-fashioned action-man surgeon that you feel something that does not exist is to invite ridicule or a psychiatric diagnosis, or perhaps a suspicion that you are about to ask for money in compensation. It is not surprising, therefore, that the entire subject tends to be as ghostly as phantoms if we look for facts in the classical literature. For example, reports of phantom breasts after mastectomy are not mentioned at all in medical literature until the 1950s. It may have been just permissible to repeat anecdotal reports about brave soldiers, but women were to be seen but not heard in serious medical literature. There are now 10 papers on the subject and all agree that some 25% of women experience phantom phenomena after the breasts are surgically removed (30). What is much more disturbing about this weird phenomenon is that it can be associated with very severe pain.

When a condition makes no sense, and especially if, as we shall see, there is no satisfactory treatment, patients and doctors feel uncomfortable in more ways than one. Such a situation provokes denial, shiftiness, and unreliable reporting. The older literature on pain in amputees resembles the literature on the diagnosis and treatment of witches. For that reason, some of us decided to make a fresh and unbiased survey of an entire group of amputees. We examined an unselected half of all the Israeli solders who suffered traumatic amputations during the 1973 Yom Kippur War, a month-long period of intense and vicious fighting (13). All amputees were admitted to a single hospital, Tel Hashomer near Tel Aviv, soon after emergency surgery was complete, and we examined 73 men with an average age of 26, ranging from 19 to 45.

This was an opportunity to reconsider Beecher's conclusions from American soldiers on the Anzio beachhead. Like his casualties, the great majority of these men reported to their surprise that their initial awareness of their injury was free of pain. We then asked them if they felt relief on being wounded, which was Beecher's explanation for the pain-free state. The situation in the Sinai and on the Golan Heights was very different from the Anzio situation. The Israelis were a few hours from their homes, rather than trapped on a beach 4000 miles from home. On further enquiry, the actual circumstances of most injuries were very different from the John Wayne–Rambo picture of blazing guns and frenzy. Many were, in fact, wounded in traffic accidents driving at full speed on hill tracks without lights. Some had been hit without warning while peacefully brewing tea, miles from the fighting. Some had indeed been fighting desperately for their lives in bunkers on the Canal, but not one spoke of relief on being wounded.

On the contrary, a surprising number blamed themselves, as had the civilians in Montreal. An example was a man who had been standing in the turret of an armored personnel carrier when he saw a wire-guided missile heading straight for it. He ducked his head into the turret but left his hands on the rim. One hand was blown off. He blamed himself for not shifting his hands instead of congratulating himself on getting his head out of the way. Most patients showed a socially admired, if misguided, stoicism and fatalism and did not use their unfortunate condition to evoke pity, public recognition, or compensation. Let us examine what happened to them.

All reported the presence of a phantom limb, 65% by the first day. Two-thirds also reported phantom pain. The pain words used were jabs, strong current, burning, knifelike, pressure, cramps, and crushing. Examination of the well-healed stumps showed patches of greatly increased sensitivity in all cases. In the wards, the shambles of the early days was replaced by a cheerful atmosphere—relatives with baskets of food, visiting delegations of schoolchildren with flowers and songs. This too passed, as did many of the pains, but not all. For some men, the pain persisted when they were out of hospital, trying to reconstruct their lives. A further survey of these men 5 to 10 years later showed that they were still in pain. Similarly, in a study of Danish women who had had a mastectomy, 3% were with phantom breast pain one month after the operation and reexamination one year later showed exactly the same percentage (30).

In America, a survey was made of 2000 military amputees in chronic pain (56, 57). Because it was suspected that military casualties might differ from civilians, the researchers compared the veterans with 436 civilians and found exactly the same picture. A careful Danish survey of older people who had elective surgical amputations of legs because they had blood vessel disease showed that over half were in pain a year later (4, 27). The saddest aspect of the situation is that 50 different types of therapy, from surgery to psychotherapy, had been tried on various patients, and none of them worked. The most obscene aspect when treatment failed was that 2% were told that nothing could be done, 5% were told that the pain would go away no matter how many years they had suffered, 24% found their questions avoided, and the rest were told it was all imaginary. Here we see impotent professionals shifting blame from their own inadequacy in an attempt to make the patient responsible. The cruel implication is not only that the problem is a mental aberration, but that a person of good character would not have invented such a preposterous symptom in the first place. Patients of every kind must be aware of the consequences of failing to respond to the miracles of modern medicine. Fortunately, the situation is improving a little as the mechanisms that generate the pain become apparent.

In the next chapter we will discuss those mechanisms in detail, but we can give a brief preview of three that relate to amputation pains. The massive nerve barrage associated with the original injury can result in a long-lasting, grumbling fire among the cells of the spinal cord. When patients have to be operated on with cool decision, this effect can be avoided, as a group of Danish doctors have shown, and pain can be prevented (4). Once nerves have been cut, they attempt to grow out seeking their former home, which is now missing. These regenerating nerves become unstable and give rise to false signals. Finally, it has been recognized that nerve damage triggers a cascade of changes, which sweeps slowly from the point of injury into the central nervous system. This cascade depends not on nerve impulses, but on chemicals that are transported by nerve fibers. The nervous system, which has lost its normal input signals, reacts by increasing its excitability in an attempt to capture whatever impulses arrive. This readjustment is overdone and results in increased sensitivity and occasional spontaneous explosions.

These new discoveries offer hope for the future, but in the meantime they offer understanding for the patient who should have received respect and sympathy in the first place. Patients need no longer hide in shame because their experiences seem to encourage the doctors' proclamation that every intractable pain is imaginary. Every amputee has more pain when upset and less when busy. Almost all report the pain worse in damp, rainy weather. We will finish this section with a true story. A very senior orthopedic surgeon who was in charge of an amputee center said, "Can you imagine it! One of the amputees told me today that his leg pain was worse when he urinated. That is fantasy for you." Had that surgeon been in closer contact with his patients, he would have known that this experience is universal among leg amputees, but they are embarrassed or frightened to mention such a bizarre observation in case they are not taken seriously.

HEADACHES, BACKACHES, AND OTHER PAINS

Amputation is (we are glad to say) an exceptional experience, but there are other extremely common pains that cannot easily be explained by injury. Let us consider headaches. Most headaches, although troublesome, are quite tolerable, and we can expect them to disappear, so we are able to ignore them. But some headaches are so painful that it is impossible to carry on with normal activity, and a bad migraine attack is among the worst experiences in the whole repertoire of pain. Rarely can we formulate a relationship between injury—if we can trace any injury at all—and the severity of the pain. Headaches are classically divided into two large groups. Tension headaches were once thought to be caused by excessive muscle contraction, but modern measurement shows little relation to muscle. The other group, vascular headache or migraine, shows even less relation to spasm of blood vessels (53).

We can identify obvious triggers of a headache: a blow on the head, loud noise, anxiety and stress, shortage of sleep, excessive consumption of alcohol. But these factors do not invariably generate a headache—certainly not for all individuals—and a headache can occur in the absence of any of them.

Low back pain is among the most widespread of pain conditions, affecting millions of people. For some of them, the pain is moderate and tolerable and goes away after a while if they continue with normal life. For others, it is agonizing and incapacitating and never goes away.

In many cases, the origin of the pain can be convincingly ascribed to a particular incident, such as bending down to pick up a heavy object, or to cumulative strain and "wear and tear" on the vertebrae. Workers in certain industries are known to be exceptionally liable to back pain. Nurses are a special example of work-induced back problems. The patient reasonably seeks comfort in the familiar low, broad bed, over which the nurse has to lean. The high, narrow modern treatment bed is kinder on the nurse's back, but the cliff-hanging posture terrifies the patient. Dame Cicely Saunders, founder of the hospice movement—we shall meet her again—is of impressive stature physically as well as intellectually. She turned from philosophy to nursing when World War II broke out and soon wrecked her back. Even today, a recent study of 66 nurses in a large Swedish hospital found that all of them had been on the sick list with back pain in the previous 2 years (31).

However, the only definite causes of back pain are herniation of discs in the spine and arthritis of vertebral joints. In a large study of patients with back pain, involving X-rays and thorough orthopedic examination, between 60% and 78% of each sample showed no sign of either of these conditions (33). Their pain had no apparent cause and was related to no detectable injury. It's no wonder that sufferers from back pain make the rounds of physicians, osteopaths, psychiatrists, and so forth in the hope of finding the "real" explanation and cure. Sadly, they often collect more theoretical knowledge than relief from pain.

Nowadays, when we cannot readily find a cause for any pain or disorder, we are inclined to say that it is psychosomatic. The word, indicating that a physical (somatic) event has a psychological determinant, has entered the vocabulary of all educated, and some not so educated, people. There is no doubt of the validity of the concept. When we are confronted with anxiety, with emotional conflict, with difficult problems, with depressing experiences or bad news, our normal condition of sound health and smooth functioning is weakened, perhaps at the most vulnerable point. [In Heine's poem, the old soldier who learns of Napoleon's defeat exclaims: *"Wie brennt meine alte Wunde!"* (*"How my old wound burns!"*).] Anxiety brings on headaches in a great many people, stomach pains and cramps in some, a variety of aches and pains in others. Some recurrent disorders—in particular, migraine, asthma, and eczema—are widely held to be triggered by stress, anxiety, and depression, and indeed often are.

It should be said, however, that to postulate a psychosomatic origin for pain whenever it occurs would be as risky— and as unscientific—as to make any other kind of automatic and invariable assumption. To admit to an anxiety when it clearly exists and can be identified is sensible and may bring peace of mind. To hunt for an anxiety without a discernible reason, simply because pain is felt, will do nothing to relieve the pain and may indeed create an anxiety that didn't exist before. We should be careful not to fall into the Cartesian error of visualizing mind and body as two separate entities, the one making an independent impact on the other. There cannot be a two-stage process of *first* the psychological problem and *then* the sensation of physical pain.

We return to the question of the relationship between injury and pain. One of the very worst pains that can be experienced is connected with the process of passing a kidney stone. If the kidney concentrates some components in the urine to form solid structures, these must pass through the ureter, which is the channel connecting the kidney to the bladder. The exceptional strain causes the muscle of the ureter to expand and contract until the process is completed. This is inevitably painful, but logic would lead us to think that the pain should be quite mild. The ureter is distended to no more than twice its normal size; the tissue damage is minor and transient; the ureter is poorly innervated, so that relatively few nerve impulses are sent to the spinal cord; and when the crisis is over, relief is immediate and complete. Why, then, should such a minor and by no means dangerous internal injury cause such terrible pain? No one knows. All that we know is that the relationship between injury and pain is out of proportion.

INJURY AND PAIN: VARIATIONS ON A THEME

We can sum up what we have learned on this subject by listing five different situations:

1. The normal situation, when injury and pain seem appropriate to each other. You cut your hand slightly and suffer a slight pain; you cut your hand badly and suffer a bad pain. The normal situation occurs so often, especially in cases of acute

pain, that most people are led into taking the common-sense view that a linear relationship between injury and pain is a universal law. We have seen that this is not so.

2. Pain is experienced without any apparent injury. The explanation may be a failure of diagnosis; i.e., an injury has occurred but cannot be detected. But, in the present state of knowledge, there are many cases in which we do not have an explanation and cannot find one even by using the most advanced diagnostic techniques.

3. Pain can be attributed to a past injury; the tissue damage healed, perhaps a long time ago, but the pain is still felt. Phantom limb pain is the most striking example of this situation, but not the only one.

4. Deafferentation pain. The pain in this case is caused by the blocking or interruption of afferent nerve impulses, rather than directly by tissue damage.

5. Finally, psychological pain is in a category of its own. An experience that the sufferer describes in terms of pain—most frequently, a headache—has its source in a purely psychological event, such as sorrow, disappointment, or humiliation. Clearly, in this situation we would look in vain for injury.

5

Mechanisms of Pain

Scientist–philosophers began the process of discovery by thinking about their own sensations; then they searched the nervous system for mechanisms that would create such sensations. They made a series of assumptions about the nature of sensations and looked for mechanisms that would fulfill the assumptions. The result is the basis of classical philosophy and science. Now a new science is appearing that depends on a reexamination of the old assumptions.

The old assumptions (hypotheses) are:

1. Sensation is subdivided into primary sensations.
2. Sensation reflects instantaneous reality.
3. Sensation is followed by perception.
4. Sensation prolonged is simply a repetition of brief sensations.

PRIMARY SENSATIONS

From the time of Democritus, the physical world was divided into a collection of indivisible particles, the atoms. The senses that reflected the physical world were similarly subdivided into separate fundamentals. First came Aristotle's five senses: vision, hearing, smell, taste, and the body sense. Just as the real world consisted of combinations of atoms, so the sensed world was made up of combinations of the primary senses.

Further introspection and experiment led to finer subdivisions of the senses. For color: from Newton through Goethe and Helmholtz, all color could be constructed from combinations of the three primary colors: red, green, and blue. For sound: all sounds could be synthesized from single frequencies (the notes), multiples (the octaves), and fractions (the harmonics). For the body sense, it seemed obvious that all sensations could be constructed from combinations of touch, warm, cool, and pain. Beyond these four there were suggestions of further primaries, such as itch and tickle, because these seemed to be so distinctive that they could not be synthesized from mixtures of the four basic primaries. Part of the growing scientific tradition was to probe each phenomenon with smaller and smaller perturbations until the indivisible particles became apparent.

By the end of the nineteenth century, examination of skin senses with tiny probes revealed that sensitivity was not uniform. Little spots could be discovered, some particularly sensitive to touch, some to warm or to cool or to pain. It seemed by this time that the classical approach was fully justified and that the skin was, in fact, a fine mosaic of detectors, with one type of detector for each of the primaries. This powerful conclusion needs particularly careful reexamination because, if true, it suggests physically separate systems for each of the primaries. Furthermore, it suggests that this separation exists as a property of skin. Before we return to this reexamination, it is necessary first to examine the decision to select pain as a primary.

EXTERNAL REALITIES AND INTERNAL REALITIES

When Aristotle listed the five senses, he was defining the ways in which we sense the world outside and around us.

Because we are highly skilled in the use of these senses, and because we share that external world with other people, we are able to talk and write about what we do through our seeing, hearing, and touching. However, there are other sensory experiences that relate to the world inside us. Examples of these sensations are hunger, thirst, and nausea. They differ from the sensations generated by external realities in several crucial ways.

We have scarcely any language to describe them (by comparison with the vast number of words whereby we describe what we see, hear, and touch). They have intensity, but no location (you cannot say just *where* you are hungry). They are always important to us (whereas a sensed external reality may be unimportant or neutral). As they grow, they can be totally dominant. And—a very significant point—they are associated with needs.

We must therefore ask the question "Does pain refer to external or internal reality?" The answer is, obviously, "both." A hypodermic needle in midair is a clearly sensed visual external reality. As the tip hits the skin, an additional sense is added, pain, which is precisely localized and described. The needle is pushed farther and becomes an internal reality. There is now no accurate sense of the location of the needle tip, and quite different sensations may be evoked depending on which structures are hit.

Some pains are associated with purely internal realities— for example, a heart attack, a twisted ankle, appendicitis, arthritis. These pains are similar to the other internal senses in that they are difficult to describe except for their intensity, and as they grow, they dominate totally. They are associated with the need for relief and recovery. However, unlike the other internal sensory experiences, these pains have a location, which is frequently referred to the surface and to a locus distant from the actual source. This referred localization of pain is a special feature of deep disease. In attempting to put words to these pains, the sufferer recruits words from the external world.

The pain of a heart attack is "a band around the chest." Phrases such as "in a vise," "pins and needles," "stabbing," "on fire," "crawling ants" all reach into the vocabulary of the outside world in order to describe internal events for which no words exist. Despite the great importance of a sentence such as "I feel a stabbing pain," the speaker is forced to use an indirect allegorical form of speech. If he were pedantically accurate, he would say, "Although I have never been stabbed and although I know I am not being stabbed now, I feel something which is what I imagine I would feel if I were stabbed." No wonder people have difficulty talking about their pains.

SENSATION REFLECTS INSTANTANEOUS REALITY

This hypothesis has played an important part in intellectual history. Philosophers such as Hume, Berkeley, and Kant were preoccupied with the problem of the relationship between reality and perception. The science of psychophysics was created to work out the relationship between the existence of an event, determined by objective physical measurement, and the existence of a sensation. Pain was clearly a case in point, so trained volunteers were subjected to pressure, heat, or electric shocks. As the intensity of the stimulus rose, they could declare a threshold and then a pain level, precisely related to the stimulus. These experiments seemed to validate the hypothesis.

It was recognized that there were obvious deviations, but these were given *ad hoc* explanations so that the general rule could be preserved. Tenderness—something that everyone has experienced—is an example of a deviation. The effect of tenderness is that pain is evoked by a gentle, innocuous stimulus. This phenomenon was explained away by deciding that the normally reliable injury–pain detectors had become pathologically sensitive. The most dramatic example of sensation failing to reflect reality is pain in a phantom limb. Here is Descartes' answer:

It is manifest that, notwithstanding the sovereign goodness of God, the nature of man, in so far as it is a composite of mind and body, must sometimes be at fault and deceptive. For should some cause, not in the foot, but in another part of the nerves that extend from the foot to the brain, or even in the brain itself, give rise to the motion ordinarily excited when the foot is injuriously affected, pain will be felt just as though it were in the foot, and thus naturally the sense will be deceived. The same motion in the brain cannot but give rise in the mind always to the same sensation. Since this sensation is much more frequently due to a cause that is injurious to the foot than by one acting in another quarter, it is reasonable that it should convey to the mind pain as in the foot.

Thus, in 1641 Descartes invented the idea of a false alarm where something has gone wrong with the signaling system. In this view, the mind is a slave of the senses, rather like an astronaut trapped in a capsule whose only contact with the world is the array of dials on the capsule wall. There is no way to tell if the readings on the dials are a true or false indication of events in the world outside. Descartes is precise and insistent on the independent and isolated nature of the mind, which is informed by the senses but which has no way of verifying and validating the senses. This is the first consequence of the separation of mind and body. That separation is called dualism.

SENSATION IS FOLLOWED BY PERCEPTION

This hypothesis, which is tightly bound to Descartes' dualism and the separation of mind and body, postulates two distinct phrases of sensory experience. The first is the consequence of a relatively mechanical reception of signals about the "true" nature of events, which results in sensation. These incidents are then perceived by the mind through a later, secondary process, which dresses up the incidents with memories, significance, predictions, and meanings.

The latter process includes the transition from sense to essence. If the sensory data include hair, teeth, nose, tail, and paws, the mind can identify them as belonging to a class of objects called dogs. The sensory data were perceived as including the essence of dogginess. The mind can construct essences, or generalizations or classes, from sets of particular sensory data. The dogginess of dogs for humans is therefore a creation of the human mind. The dogginess of dogs for dogs is a creation of the dog's mind. (Descartes was not British and denied that dogs had minds. For him, they were purely sensory mechanical creatures.)

Applying this hypothesis to pain, one should be aware first of the data as pure sensory pain. This should be followed by a mental and conscious perception in which the pure pain is dressed in its clothes of meaning and misery. The mind is by definition clever, certainly clever enough to give the pain a location. If you pick up a telephone and hear, "This is Mary Smith calling from New York," you do not stop to think that the actual origin of the sound is in the earpiece. You accept signals as originating from a distant place. Similarly, you classify signals into general groups and give them names such as pain. This involves grouping together very different signals such as a pinprick or appendicitis or even "purely psychological pain," for example, the death of a friend, which is classed as the equivalent of a personal injury.

SENSATION PROLONGED IS A REPETITION OF BRIEF SENSATIONS

Since the mechanical reporting of the sensory system was thought of as the minute-by-minute action of reliable signaling machinery, there was traditionally no need to differentiate between acute and chronic pain. When a patient reported a sensation of pain, he must have been reporting the arrival of signals provoked by injury. If a patient reported pain without an appropriate injury, then it must have been an invention of an aberrant mind, to be treated accordingly. Such was the accepted view both of philosophers and of medical practitioners.

HYPOTHESES AND MECHANISMS

Scientists, however, were under an obligation to find and describe mechanisms that would support the four hypotheses outlined above. Let us look first at the mechanisms related to primary sensations.

As we have seen, traditional thought gave little, if any, intellectual respect to the senses. A simple mechanical reporting system was all they were allowed; all subtlety or cleverness was a property of the mind. Sensory mechanisms could therefore be visualized as little more than the equivalent of fire-alarm or burglar-alarm systems.

The nineteenth century was a busy time for clinicians and scientists in their progressive exploration of the brain. It began with a considerable argument between those who thought of the brain as an indivisible whole and those who thought that it must be subdivided into separate specialized parts. The subdividers won the argument and set about a geographical exercise in which the intention was to make maps of the brain with a functional label assigned to each delineated zone. By the end of the century, Ramón y Cajal had shown that the brain was made up of separate units, the nerve cells. The ultimate ambition of the map makers was to assign a single function to each cell. The clinicians who became particularly concerned with brain function formed into a distinct group, the neurologists. At the same time, following the age of reason, some medical men began to think of mental functions in terms of brain function. Thus, the specialty of psychiatry appeared. Although such heresy no longer carried the danger of being burned at the stake, these new doctors were careful to preserve dualism. The neurologists were free to study the mechanical functions of brain and sensation, while the psychiatrists could hint at the more doubtful and dangerous proposal that at least some mental aberrations had a material basis in malfunction of the brain.

The frontier between the mind and the body had to be defended in bitter battles, which continue today between the warring battalions of the two professions, with their support troops of priests, psychologists, computer engineers, and philosophers. An example of such a battle is the analysis of a *grand mal* epileptic seizure. It can begin with an aura, brilliantly described in *The Idiot* by Dostoyevsky, who was himself an epileptic. In this stage of epilepsy there may be a huge mood change, with periods of exaltation, brilliant visions, and enhanced powers of prediction and understanding. These seemingly meaningful mental events merge with a predictable progression of mechanical body movements. The whole sequence is accompanied by detectable electrical changes, which can be measured by the electroencephalograph. It is easy to see how the two sides have become confused as to which side they are fighting on and what they are fighting about. The Arab–Israeli conflict is simple by comparison, although here too, it is hard to dissociate a single definable issue from a mountain of history, belief, religion, and philosophy.

The clinical neurologists began to notice and report localized lesions in the human brain associated with specific deficits. The career of one of these pioneers, a physician named Franz Josef Gall (1757–1828), is revealing. He was expelled from Catholic Austria for the heresy of maintaining that the physical organ called the brain generates the mind. Not content with this, he showed that people with localized tumors and localized injuries had localized problems with their sensations and with the movement of particular limbs. He used this as evidence against those who believed the brain to be a unitary whole. At this point he began to err in two respects. The first was the question of how to label the parts. Gall picked on categories such as hope, calculation, love, and language. He was right about language, because local destruction of small parts of the brain does lead to aphasia, or inability to speak. He was wrong about his other categories, which were really selected by the same introspective guesswork that led to the sensory primaries.

Gall's second aberration has, in retrospect, an element of black humor. He noticed that bumps on the skull reflected bumps on the brain, particularly when slow-growing tumors (meningiomas) existed on the surface of the brain. He therefore concluded that inspection of the brain itself was quite unnecessary, because the relative size of all the areas could be deduced by feeling (palpating) the bumps on the skull. This led to the mid-nineteenth-century fascination with the pseudoscience of phrenology, which persists today not only in the shape of beautiful porcelain bald heads to be found in antique shops, but also as the basis for a school of alternative medicine, cranial osteopathy.

Phrenology made no headway in devoutly Catholic countries, such as Gall's own Austria, because it conflicted with the established concept of the soul. However, in Western societies, which accorded high esteem to science (or anything that claimed to be science), it spread like wildfire. America was particularly enthusiastic. Institutes of phrenology were set up in all major American cities, illnesses were confidently diagnosed, and companies sent job applicants to have their character assessed as a guide to their suitability for employment. Needless to say, the medical establishment labeled all this as charlatan quackery, forgetting that it originated from perfectly correct and repeatable observation.

What precisely was right and what was wrong with this approach to the brain? Napoleon made an astonishingly perceptive statement about Gall: "He ascribes to certain prominences of the skull, propensities and crimes which do not exist in nature but are the growth of society and are merely conventional. What would the organ of theft effect, if there were no property? What would the organ of drunkenness do if there were no liquor, or the organ of ambition if there were no society?" Napoleon was asking exactly the right questions without doubting the facts of localization. Had Gall selected the right primary brain functions? Could they exist in isolation? These are exactly the questions to be considered for sensation in general and pain in particular.

The first major step in defining sensory mechanisms was the discovery that the sensory information from the body to the brain and spinal cord flowed in anatomically separate channels, the dorsal roots. This crucial observation is attributed by some to Sir Charles Bell (1774–1842). His name is remembered in Bell's palsy, the condition in which one side of the face is suddenly and completely paralyzed although sensitivity remains intact. His writings are rather vague on the explanation of this separation of sensory nerves from motor nerves. There are those who claim he changed his early writing when the discovery was made in full clarity by François Magendie (1783–1855). In any case, these pioneers were unpopular with their contemporaries. One wrote of Magendie's *Journal of Physiology*: "It is the kind of journal one would expect from a man who works alone and who separates himself voluntarily from collaborators whose talent would dim his own star." Yet Magendie's discovery was crucial, not only because it gave a location to part of the sensory mechanism, but—even more important—because it led to the idea of direction of flow. Sensory signals (the input) arrive over the dorsal roots, while motor signals, which produce movement (the output), leave over the ventral roots. Quite apart from the location of sensory input, the discovery provided an anatomical structure for the reflex arc. The reflex, a stimulus followed by a response, was itself to become one of the fundamental building blocks from which anatomists and physiologists were to construct the units of behavior. (See Fig. 4.)

The next stage was to subdivide the sensory inputs. This was clearly proposed by Johannes Petrus Muller (1801–1858), who said that there must be five sensory inputs with their associated sensory brains, one for each of the Aristotelian five senses. Each brain must have a "specific energy," the nature of which was not specified. There followed a scramble to identify the structures associated with the five senses and those which were responsible for movement. Descartes' termination of "delicate threads" in the pineal gland was abandoned in favor of interrupted pathways that ran from the sense organs through various stages to terminate in the primary sensory areas of the cerebral cortex. (See Figs. 7 and 8.)

Technical advances played an essential part in this search. Staining methods using dyes and new microscopes allowed single cells and anatomical pathways to be identified. The discovery of "animal electricity" by Galvani and Volta led to the possibility of artificially stimulating selected parts of the brain and recording the naturally occurring electrical activity, i.e., the nerve impulses. With the development of anesthesia and antiseptic surgery, animals could be subjected to specific damage in imitation of human diseases. Thus, surgical excision of the cortex of a monkey reproduced the effect of a stroke, paralyzing

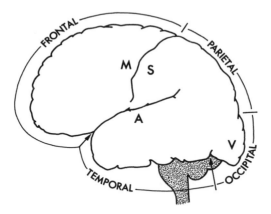

FIGURE 7. The cerebral cortex seen from one side. There are four large lobes: frontal, parietal, occipital, and temporal. The motor cortex (M) lies in front of the central fissure that separates the frontal from the parietal lobe. Sensory information from the body arrives in the cortex at S from the eyes at V and from the ears at A.

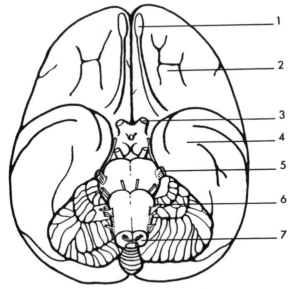

FIGURE 8. The brain seen from below. (1) The olfactory nerves supplied from the nose; (2) the bottom surface of the frontal lobes; (3) the optic nerves from the eyes; (4) the bottom surface of the temporal lobes; (5) the trigeminal nerve, sensory nerve from the face; (6) the auditory nerve, sensory nerve from the ears; (7) the spinal cord.

the animal's arm. When this monkey was shown to Jean-Martin Charcot (1825–1893), a key founder of neurology and psychiatry, he made the pontifical pronouncement: "C'est un malade" ("It is a sick person"). The word *malade* would normally be applied only to a human being. The historic achievement was to lead to an explanation of how men and women have strokes.

At the same time, the impact of Darwin's discovery of evolution was affecting all thinking about living creatures, and nowhere so fundamentally as in thinking about the brain. If species evolved one from another, so also did the parts of the species. If behavior evolved, so did the brain responsible for the behavior. By comparing the brains of animals, it should be possible to locate those newly evolved parts which are responsible for newly evolved behaviors. If brains, from a worm's brain to a human brain, are compared, there is a very obvious steady advance with an increasing proportion of nerve tissue within the head. Among the vertebrates and certainly among the mammals, the plan of the spinal cord and that of the medulla oblongata, or hindbrain, are remarkably similar. There is, however, a huge progressive increase in the relative size and complexity of the forebrain, particularly of the cerebral cortex. Even comparing monkeys, apes, and humans, there is a further exaggeration of the size of the cerebral cortex and its associated inputs.

Herbert Spencer, the polymath who introduced the phrase "the survival of the fittest," strongly influenced the neurologist Hughlings Jackson (1835–1911), among the first to think of the brain in evolutionary terms. From this came the idea of higher and lower levels of the nervous system. The highest level associated with the highest, most recently evolved functions was the cerebral cortex. The lowest, oldest level was the spinal cord. Jackson compared the organization of the brain to the largest, most complex, most successful organization he knew, the Royal Navy. The ordinary seamen inhabited the spinal cord, connected through a hierarchical chain of command to the Board of Admiralty, housed in the cerebral cortex. His analogy was more subtle than this Gilbert-and-Sullivan image might imply. For example, the loss of a group of seamen caused an irrevocable failure of part of the system, the equivalent of anesthesia or paralysis. If an admiral died, the other admirals on the Board just took over and did his job and the organization continued. However, if one admiral went mad, there could be serious consequences with which the rest of the Board could not cope.

Manipulate the facts or the analogies as you will, a very serious and definite conclusion had been reached by the brain scientists. They found it entirely logical to locate the machinery of sensation and perhaps perception in the cerebral cortex.

Each of the five senses had its primary sensory area in the cortex (Fig. 7). The body sense had its special area within which the entire surface of the body was precisely mapped. Let us emphasize that the anatomical, physiological, and neurological facts are true facts. It is the location of psychological function in these areas which is not a fact but a hypothesis. But that hypothesis became so accepted that it was taken to be a fact.

The stage was now set to continue the subdivision of the body senses and to identify and label the separate mechanisms of the primaries. This was apparently achieved in 1894 and 1895 by Max von Frey in a remarkable series of papers that bring together three approaches. The first was the intuitive subdivision into the four primaries: touch, warm, cool, and pain. The second was to use tiny probes and to show that there were particularly sensitive spots on the skin, one type for each primary. The third approach was a great leap of the imagination. Anatomists were by that time able to stain cells and nerve fibers and had found that some sensory nerve fibers end in elaborate special structures with a clear form. von Frey proposed that under each sensitive spot, one of these structures would be found and would be the anatomical label explaining why that piece of skin was particularly sensitive to touch or warm or cool. He also saw that some nerve ends just terminate as bare ends without any protective covering, like the twigs of a tree in winter. To these he assigned pain.

What could be simpler, more attractive, and more in the spirit of the times? The reader is warned that the primary sensations, the sensitive spots, and the nerve ends are facts, but the linkages between them are hypotheses. However, the hypotheses became accepted as facts. The trouble was that in the course of all this indubitable progress, an error had crept in. This was the supposition that since there were nerve fibers carrying signals of pressure, heat, or cold, there must be other nerve fibers whose specific function was to transmit pain. (In analyzing this supposition, we shall call it the specificity theory.) The idea of a "pain pathway" became generally acceptable and led to a corollary—the idea of a specific "pain center" in the brain.

Only later did it occur to scientists to ask why the sensation of pain was not transmitted with the same invariable accuracy as heat or cold—why individuals gave evidence of more, or sometimes less, pain than they ought to have felt. The pain pathway, therefore, came under scrutiny. After some 30 years of intensive research, nothing resembling a specialized system of pain nerves could be found. Nor was a pain center found.

Meanwhile, scientists equipped with newly developed techniques were investigating single nerve fibers leading from the skin to the spinal cord (as described earlier). They found two classes of fiber sensitive to injury. These nociceptors are the small myelinated fibers, the A-delta fibers, and the even smaller unmyelinated fibers, the C fibers.

In order to complete this updated version of the Descartes picture, it was now only necessary to determine the link between the peripheral nerve fibers and the cerebral cortex. It was found that the nociceptive fibers terminated and relayed onto nerve cells soon after entering the spinal cord. How did these cells send signals to the cerebral cortex? This question was apparently answered by the early years of this century. The overcrowded slums of the nineteenth century had produced the mass epidemic of tuberculosis. In one late, untreated stage of this disease, small, hard, round lumps, called tuberculomas, can grow anywhere in the body. If they grow on the spinal cord, the result is destruction of part of the spinal cord. When the front (anterior or ventral) part of the cord was destroyed on one side, neurologists observed the astonishing fact that the patient could not detect pinpricks, pinches, or heat on the *other* side of the body, though light touch was reported quite accurately. Similar cases of one-sided analgesia (inability to feel pain) were found in people who had survived stabs in the back with stilettoes. Just such a case was seen by W. H. Spiller in 1905, and he began to wonder if these accidents of disease or assault could be intentionally imitated by neurosurgeons for the benefit of patients in pain. By 1911, at his instigation, Martin carried out that operation. This was the origin of the cordotomy operation as a remedy for pain. Among the nerve fibers cut in the operation, some run directly from the spinal cord to the thalamus, where they relay and project to the cortex. What had been achieved was to give modern labels to the "delicate threads" that transmitted pain in Descartes' model:

1. Stage 1: Peripheral nerve fibers (A-delta or C fibers)
2. Stage 2: Dorsal horn cells projecting by way of the opposite ventral spinal cord
3. Stage 3: Thalamus
4. Stage 4: Cortex

MECHANISMS FOR THE OTHER HYPOTHESES

Once it was generally accepted that the mechanisms for the sensation of pain had been identified and located, it was easy to fit the other hypotheses into this framework. The intensity of the sensation of pain in trained subjects could be shown to reflect the intensity of a stimulus that damaged (or threatened to damage) tissue. True, some of these trained volunteers had to be dismissed as unreliable witnesses because they gave the wrong answers, while ordinary people were quite useless.

There were three ways of dealing with people whose reports of pain (or absence of pain) failed to reflect the amount of injury. The simplest was to dismiss such reports as unreliable. The second was Descartes' way, suggesting that a faulty signaling system could generate false signals. The third and favorite method was to attribute all aberrations to mental processes that failed to announce correctly the state of incoming sensory signals. Ordinary folk could be neglected because they were not paying proper attention and did not understand what was required of them. Even among trained subjects, it had to be admitted that some would cease reporting pain when they were given a placebo. These were put in a special class called "placebo reactors," which, like a psychiatric diagnosis, meant that they were subject to fantasy states that went against common sense. A new phrase, "nociceptive pain," was introduced. It indicated pain appropriate to the amount of injury and the presence of nerve impulses in sensory afferent nociceptors. All other pains or absence of pains were explained as false signals or as mental aberrations.

Thus, dualism reigned. Most neuroscientists contended themselves with a search for pure sensory mechanisms and fought shy of seeking mechanisms for perception. The very word "perception" (let alone "self-consciousness," "intention," and "meaning") was put aside as either meaningless or not yet a proper subject for scientific investigation. Even the psychologists withdrew to a straightforward study of stimulus and behavioral response without speculation about the nature of any intervening mental processes. Although dualism was accepted as a fact, it was, curiously, not investigated.

Yet even Descartes had written: "External objects are able to impress the soul." This statement challenges the dualistic scientist at least to define where and how this impression takes place. Sir John Eccles, the Australian who won a Nobel Prize for his work on the nervous system, took up this challenge along with the philosopher Sir Karl Popper. Eccles wrote:

> The unity of conscious experience is provided by the self-conscious mind and not by the neural machinery of the liaison areas of the cerebral hemispheres. . . . The self-conscious mind can scan the activity of each module of the liaison brain or at least those modules tuned to its present interest. . . . The self-conscious mind has the function of integrating its selections from the immense patterned input it receives from the liaison brain . . . in order to build its experiences from moment to moment.

The reader will immediately see that these fine words only define and locate the frontier between two worlds. The sensory world terminates precisely in the cerebral cortex as a collection of isolated modules. Beyond is a quite separate world, which retreats like a will-o'-the-wisp. While appearing to add a modern precision to the meaning and nature of mind–body relations, Eccles and Popper were vituperative about a small opposing school, the monists. The monists consider that the brain is an integrated whole and that a separation of sensation from perception is an intellectual trick resulting from excessive introspective attempts at orderly subdivision of the indivisible. Eccles and Popper label monists as simple-minded mechanists who deny any of the engaging qualities of humankind and see the human being as nothing but a mass of interlocked gear wheels. This is really a case of the pot calling the kettle black. Dualists like Eccles and Popper describe a deterministic body machinery performing its mechanical ordained task, observed by a conscious mind full of ideas, feelings, and emotions. By assigning all the glories of humanity to an unobservable mind, it is they who trivialize the body machinery.

Such was the situation reached by the second half of the twentieth century. Then new facts began to appear that challenged the old assumptions.

NEW FACTS AND THEIR IMPLICATIONS

"There is nothing new under the sun" applies as much in science as in other spheres. By midcentury the life sciences were set on a very specific course, which aimed to collapse all of biology into biochemistry and beyond biochemistry into molecular biology. An enormous step along that path was the identification of the nature of DNA by James Watson and Francis Crick as the molecule that contained the coded instructions on how to build cells and whole animals. Once the time arrived when the mass of blueprint instructions would be reduced to individual orders, it seemed that there would be no logical or even practical reasons why the analytical process should not be turned around in order to build or synthesize whatever was desired. Watson, a powerful advocate of this reductionist approach, said: "There are only atoms. Everything else is merely social work."

To achieve this process, it is obviously crucially important to pick some clearly isolated and isolatable whole in order to atomize it into its components. This requirement made pain mechanisms, as classically described, a particularly attractive target because if pain fibers, pathways, and centers had been identified and isolated, it remained necessary only to work in the hugely powerful new techniques of molecular biology to identify the "specific nerve energies" for pain as molecules. This path is being followed by many neuroscientists. It is important to emphasize that even if this singular specific path is a blind alley, they will find many fascinating and important facts by serendipity.

While the development of the specificity theory of pain mechanisms was in progress, there were—needless to say—those who doubted. Psychologists mocked at the selection of pain as an isolated single primary sense (9, 60). They knew that experiments that claimed to prove this were planned on a circular design which could hardly go wrong. The brain is a marvelously plastic and obliging structure. If you ask the brain, "Are you like a computer?" it will say, "Yes. Watch me compute." However, if you ask the brain, "Are you like any existing computer?" it will retort, "Show me one as good as even the brain of a mouse."

It was the clinicians who developed the greatest challenge to von Frey's specificity theory. They saw that it simply did not explain what they learned from patients. Albert Goldscheider in 1894 decided that von Frey was wrong because he knew, for example, that some patients felt a warm test tube initially as warm and then, seconds later, as very hot and eventually as unbearably burning (23).

Four later clinicians had a particular influence on the work done in our own times by Ronald Melzack, a psychologist, and

Patrick D. Wall, a physiologist and one of the co-authors of this book. William Livingstone showed that no amount of manipulation of specific pain peripheral fibers could explain the troubles of people with nerve injuries (32). J. J. Bonica recognized acute and chronic pain as different problems (7). Henry K. Beecher had observed the paradoxically pain-free casualties on the Anzio beachhead. In 1959 he wrote a key book, *The Measurement of Subjective Responses* (6). Finally, William Noordenbos, Professor of Neurosurgery in Amsterdam, wrote a book in the same year which hammered home the bankruptcy of the idea that there was a single rigid pain mechanism (52). Another reason for the challenge made by the clinicians was the utter sterility of the specificity theory. It was unable either to explain observed pain or to generate new therapies.

This was the general situation by 1960, but Melzack and Wall, working at the Massachusetts Institute of Technology, had two advantages that allowed them to challenge the specificity theory. The first was purely technical. Electronics had advanced rapidly, and it became possible to record the activity of individual nerve cells. This allowed direct examination of the firmest prediction of the specificity theory, namely, that specialized sensory cells would be discovered that only signaled the presence of injury, and that they would do this in a reliable, fixed manner. We will discuss below the new results that made it necessary to think again about mechanisms.

The other aspect of the situation that encouraged new ways of thinking was a surge of interest in how communication occurs. This was stimulated both by the technology of electronic communication networks, which led to Claude Shannon's "information theory," and by consideration of speech itself, led by Noam Chomsky's work on grammar. As with sensation, it became apparent that the analytical subdivision of speech into its fundamental particles, the phonemes, did not lead automatically to the synthesis of grammar and semantics.

On the senses, Jerome Lettvin, Walter Pitts, and Warren McCulloch of MIT had written a paper with the bizarre title

"What the Frog's Eye Tells the Frog's Brain." This work, based on new recording techniques and new thinking, contradicted the old belief that the eye was nothing but a mosaic array of point light detectors which projected a precise image of the visible world into the brain. Instead, they showed that the visual system filtered out from the mass of detail those objects which were biologically important to the frog: moving flies, herons' beaks, and so on. This discovery raised the question of whether these event detectors were built-in, rigid, hard-wired filters or whether they might be tunable to detect particular events relevant to the particular situation. Pattern recognition, which we and animals manage so superbly, was a property that engineers wanted to build into machines. They too were faced with the alternative of making rigid hard-wired gadgets or smart soft-wired machines that could trim their circuitry to solve first one problem and then another as the demands of the situation changed.

In work undertaken in the 1960s, Melzack examined the psychology of the somatic senses while Wall concentrated on the actual physiology of the pathways. Together, they were aiming at a new theory of pain that would explain facts for which the specificity theory could not account. These facts can be summarized thus: (1) The relationship between injury and pain is variable. (2) Innocuous stimuli can produce pain. (3) The location of pain may be different from the location of damage. (4) Pain may persist in the absence of injury or after healing. (5) The nature of pain changes over time. (6) There is no adequate treatment for certain types of pain, and some of them have no ascertainable cause.

Logic required the hypothesis of a mechanism that would permit these phenomena; what remained was the task of discovering the mechanism. In 1965, it was given the name "gate control" (42). The metaphor was appropriate because a gate can be wide open, firmly closed, partially open, or open and closed at different times.

We proceed now to describe in detail the mechanisms

known to govern the experience of pain, beginning with gate control—the most important—and going on to others.

MECHANISM 1: GATE CONTROL

The mechanism in which nerve impulses enter the spinal cord and proceed to the brain comprises five stages. The following are the five stages we used in developing the original model. (See Fig. 9.)

Stage A

The small (S), myelinated A-delta fibers and the unmyelinated C fibers are stimulated by injury. They deliver impulses, directly and indirectly, to transmission (T) cells in the spinal cord that transmit to local reflex circuits and to the brain. This stage incorporates all aspects of Descartes' concept of pain.

Stage B

No synaptic junctions in the central nervous system are as simple as that shown in stage A. All synaptic regions include cells that facilitate and inhibit the flow of impulses. It was necessary to propose that there are facilitatory cells in the region of the T cells because it was known that all cells in the dorsal horn of the spinal cord fire a prolonged burst of impulses after the arrival of a brief input volley (69). Furthermore, if this volley is repeated at regular intervals, the afterdischarge becomes more and more prolonged (44, 45). The afterdischarge and its "windup" led us to incorporate an excitatory interneuron in the basic diagram, shown here as a black circle.

Stage C

Early recordings from cells in the spinal cord revealed cells that not only responded to the small, high-threshold fibers (5),

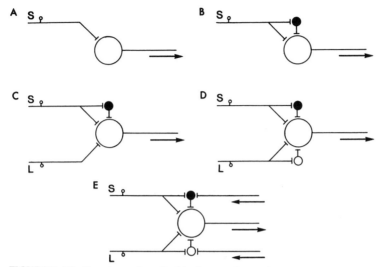

FIGURE 9. The five stages described in the text that make the final model E of the gate control.

but were also excited by large, low-threshold myelinated afferent fibers (L). Later work showed that these cells with both L and S inputs were by far the most common of the centrally projecting cells that signal injury (38, 70, 75). Because these cells respond to light pressure on the skin and increase their frequency of response as the pressure stimulus rises in intensity to a strong pinch, they have been called wide-dynamic-range (WDR) cells (44). A minority of cells are not excited by low-level stimuli and respond only when smaller afferent fibers are stimulated. These are called nociceptive-specific (NS) cells. A third group of cells respond only to low-intensity pressure stimuli. The specificity theorists concentrated on the NS cells as the only cells that could be involved in triggering pain. We, on the other hand, simply proposed that pain would be triggered if the firing rate of any group of cells exceeded a critical level determined by the properties of the brain. Much of the detailed work since 1965 has concentrated on the sensory roles of the WDR and NS cells. When we discuss new developments in the theory, we will see that the most recent results support our original proposal in unexpected ways.

Stage D

Generally, all synaptic regions contain both inhibitory and excitatory mechanisms, which control transmission depending on the balance of their activity. The inhibitory cells are shown in Figure 9 as open circles, while the facilitating cells are shown as filled circles. It was found that large-diameter afferents can inhibit as well as excite the T cells (70).

Stage E

It had long been known that powerful influences descend from the brain and modulate spinal reflexes (58). Later, it was shown that these descending effects also changed sensory messages traveling from the cord to the brain (25). Furthermore, it was shown that local stimulation in the midbrain and medulla inhibits the firing of T cells (64). Also, there was evidence that a powerful, steady inhibition flowed continually from the brain stem onto T cells (70). It was therefore reasonable to include a descending influence on the inhibitory and excitatory inter-neurons.

Finally, we assumed that ascending messages to the brain can influence the descending controls, thereby completing a loop from spinal cord to brain and back to the spinal cord.

Development of the Gate Control Theory

A five-stage model of this variety had been developed by 1965, but a great deal has happened since. The relationship between pain and the firing of nociceptors can now be studied in humans (72). That relationship varies even in highly trained volunteer subjects, depending on the situation and on the exact training. There is little relation between the time course of firing and of pain. Identical pains can be produced by very different inputs. Certainly in pathological situations such as tenderness, pain may follow activation of low-threshold afferents. In other words, the intensity, time course, and nature of pain depend on decisions in the brain and spinal cord and are not simply triggered by activity in a particular type of sensory afferent fiber. There is no possibility of a simple straight-through transmitting cell.

There has been a considerable search for the small control cells, particularly the inhibitory cells, which would be expected to decrease pain. In this field, the most exciting discovery was that narcotics were being produced by the nervous system itself and were particularly concentrated in the spinal cord exactly among the small cells at the gate entry point of incoming nerves. Two types of endogenous opiates, called enkephalins and dynorphins, are produced in the region. This discovery led not only to an understanding of why narcotics are analgesics, but to a new way of administering opiates directly onto the spinal cord, where they produce analgesia without any of the general psychedelic effects of narcotics. In addition to endogenous narcotics, the local small cells produce other chemicals, each of which opens up an opportunity for new types of pain control.

The first practical test of gate-control inhibition was the development of transcutaneous electrical nerve stimulations (TENS) (73). As we shall describe later, gentle electrical stimulation of peripheral nerves is sufficient only to stimulate the large low-threshold A-Beta fibers. The patient feels a buzzing and tingling in the area of pain, and many pains are reduced to tolerable levels. This has now become a widespread treatment. It depends on the paradoxical observation that adding one type of nerve impulse can inhibit the effects of other impulses.

Descending controls have been an obvious target for much of the later work. Different parts of the brain intrude on the transmission pathways in various subtle ways. The brain is not the passive slave of injected sensory messages. It permits penetration of those messages which it requires for its overall function and rejects those which are irrelevant. Mechanisms were found by which the brain actively selects its input second by second. As work progressed, it became apparent that there were at least two other mechanisms beyond the rapidly acting gate control.

MECHANISM 2: IMPULSE-TRIGGERED PROLONGED PAIN MECHANISMS

During the course of studies designed to unravel the stages of the gate control, a new phenomenon was observed. If the small, unmyelinated afferents, the C fibers, were made to generate a brief burst of nerve impulses, they necessarily set off immediate activity in the transmission cells, depending on the setting of the gate control. However, it was noticed that long after this burst of activity, there was a slow onset of increased excitability, which then lasted for a very long time. It was found that this was a special ability of C fibers that came from deep tissue such as joints, muscles, and internal organs but was not a property of fibers from skin. It appeared that these C fibers were releasing some special kind of chemical, which seemed to be in the family called peptides, which are naturally occurring molecules made up of short chains of amino acids. There is also evidence that this long latency and long-lasting lighting up of the system could also be accomplished by pathways descending from the brain.

The discovery of these prolonged central changes may explain some important types of pain. Twisting an ankle is acutely painful and is followed by a deep-spreading, poorly localized ache and widespread tenderness. The later phase is likely to be caused by this second mechanism. During a surgical operation, the spinal cord receives a massive bombardment of which the patient is unaware because he is unconscious. This bombardment may leave its trace in the form of increased excitability. There is now evidence that some postoperative pain is the consequence of this long-smoldering fire left over from the initial bombardment. Similarly, some pains may be "memories" of past events rather than a report of a moment-by-moment arrival of new signals. These are hopeful developments, because it may be possible to damp down these long-term traces with chemicals that do not interfere with the normal functioning of the nerve cells.

MECHANISM 3: TRANSPORT-CONTROLLED PROLONGED PAIN MECHANISMS

This mechanism operates in parallel with the gate-control and the impulse-triggered control mechanisms. The main facts are:

1. When a peripheral nerve is cut, a cascade of changes sweeps centrally during the ensuing days and weeks which alters the chemistry and physiology of the dorsal root ganglion cells, the motor neurons, and the central terminals of the sensory fibers.
2. Changes in the afferents induce changes in the spinal cord, which include a reduction of inhibitions, a spread of receptive fields, and an increase of excitability.
3. The delayed peripheral and central changes are not produced by nerve impulses because they are not altered by prolonged impulse blockade.
4. The time course and other properties of the central change support the proposal that they are produced by changes in chemicals transported within the axons of sensory fibers. Because most of the changes can be reduced by the specific C-fiber poison capsaicin, it is

believed that the unmyelinated afferents play a particularly important role.

5. The chemicals and their messages remain unknown, but nerve growth factor is a prominent candidate.

This brief summary of extensive work by many researchers introduces a new dimension to pain mechanisms. It relates to the special pains associated with peripheral nerve and dorsal root injury. The first hints of this axon transport mechanism came from the observation that the central consequences of a crushed nerve are different from those of a cut nerve. In a sense, the spinal cord seemed to "diagnose" the nature of the injury, even though peripheral axons are equally interrupted in both lesions. It was recently discovered that when C fibers are forced to grow into a new type of tissue, they take on the characteristics of the new tissue and change their central actions accordingly. This discovery tells us that C fibers are continually sensitive to the type of tissue in which they end and suggests that they detect, by chemical means, not only the existence of grossly pathological tissue but subtle variations, including the presence of normal tissue transplanted to the "wrong" place. This would give C fibers the role of "chemical pathologist," reporting that all is well or that deviations from the normal are occurring. Peripheral abnormality detected by C fibers and signaled by a change of chemical transport could result in attempts by the central nervous system to compensate for the peripheral abnormality. This could obviously play an important role in pain mechanisms.

These changed chemicals increase the excitability of the spinal cord region in which the nerve fibers end. This has the effect of increasing the ongoing activity of the transmitting cells and brings into powerful action the normally weak distant inputs, which are still intact. This mechanism could be particularly important with regard to deafferentation pains, characterized by damage to afferent sensory nerves, in cases of amputation and neuralgia.

HOW DO THESE NEW DISCOVERIES
AFFECT THE OLD ASSUMPTIONS?

By way of a summary, we can now return to reexamine the four old hypotheses. The first of these assumes that there is a discrete, unique property of injured tissue that is reflected in the sensation of pain. We have surely given enough examples of the variable link between injury and pain to make this hypothesis untenable. Furthermore, scientific research has failed to find a hard-wired system dedicated purely to detecting injury and provoking pain. Many of the experiments that purported to support the hypothesis were planned recursively so that artificial categories emerged. Imagine that a crazy general said, "There are only two types of soldiers, heroes and cowards. We give the heroes medals and put the cowards in prison. You can check on the accuracy of my statement by observing that some of my soldiers have medals and the rest are in prison." His facts might be correct, but one would see that he had made a subjective division that said nothing about the real nature of soldiers, heroes or cowards. So it is with the categorization of nerve fibers.

Let us take the apparently hard fact that detailed examination of the skin with tiny probes reveals spots sensitive to touch or warmth or cooling or pain. The simplest exact repetition of this observation shows that the spots are meandering around minute by minute, so that they cannot possibly represent the endings of nerve fibers. Furthermore, if you apply a tiny heated probe to the skin, it provokes a pain, but if you keep the temperature the same and make the probe a little larger, it feels hot; make it larger still and the feeling is pleasantly warm. Heroes and cowards, pain systems and warm systems can change dramatically depending on the situation.

We have also, we trust, said enough to make the reader doubt the unique singularity of pain as a single sensation. There are multiple pain systems, which differ in time, space, affect, and meaning. They may be loosely grouped together as an odious class known as pain, but do they reflect an instantaneous reality (the second hypothesis)? A young woman Israeli army officer with a leg blown off in an explosion was in no immediate pain but asked the immensely sad question, "Who is going to marry me now?" Her situation and her feelings changed with time. Two years later she was married but suffered severe burning pain in her stump and phantom limb. What is the reality reflected in these different situations? We have spoken of internal feelings as reflecting need states as much as injury. What was her overwhelming need in the period immediately after injury? Certainly the need to care for her comrades and to assure rapid transport out of danger to hospital received first priority. Pain was irrelevant until the need to assure the best tactics for treatment and recovery permitted the appearance of pain. Why was she in pain 2 years later when all signs of the injury had healed? The nervous system, attempting to compensate for missing incoming sensory signals, had raised its excitability within the spinal cord and brain stem and was generating insistent false signals. If she were to encounter some dramatic situation demanding a new priority of action, her pain state would once again fall into the background.

The third hypothesis presented a division between a simple reporting system and a "clever" conscious system in the mind. Reality does not validate this intellectual abstraction. To register a pure sensation, and then to bring the mind into action to decide how unpleasant it is, would be an experience no one has ever had. If pain appears at all, it appears as a loathsome package. Later reflection may help us to decide that it is dangerous or trivial, but that is another matter. The concept of a double system in which perception follows experience is supported neither by common sense nor by scientific knowledge.

Even the most devout dualist must admit that the conscious mind is not necessarily involved in the intricate complexity of human perceptions. A car driver conversing with a passenger may be quite unaware of his weaving in and out of traffic and would be unable to describe his actions afterward. A pianist playing a concerto would be a performing disaster if he consciously awaited the conductor's baton and listened for particular notes from the rest of the orchestra, even though his playing shows that he has received those signals. Clearly, the motorist or the pianist could consciously attend to the relevant events, but in the real situation they did not do this. The key word is "attend." As a prerequisite of perception by the conscious mind, attention must be attracted. But what attracts attention in the first place? It is rarely directed by a conscious effort. Normally, some unconscious brain process is sifting through the repertoire of possible priorities and either directing behavior or, on rare special occasions, directing conscious verbal analysis.

Pain appears as a perceived package after the attentional mechanisms have decided it is relevant. It does not appear first as a pure pain, after which the conscious mind directs one's attention and analytical processes to decide what to think about this pure sensation. It is true that a trained volunteer, assured that a test stimulus is not going to injure him, can be directed to attend to various aspects of the stimulus. With our clever brains, we can dissect out some aspects of our mental process. But this does not mean that it is a fundamental step in our normal feeling.

Finally, we can refute the fourth hypothesis by showing that the nervous system is a mobile reactive mechanism that shifts with circumstance and with time. The flow of consciousness is not fed by a stream of ticker-tape reporting the news moment by moment. The sensory nervous system reflects on the past as well as the present. The present is not perceived as isolated events, no matter how large and persistent they may be, but is perceived in context. The pinprick of a dentist giving a local anesthetic is sense-perceived as a different event from an identical stimulus applied by a police interrogator. We have described neural mechanisms in tissue and in the spinal cord and brain that generate a sequence of pains as time goes by. These mechanisms explain one way that acute pains can evolve into chronic pains. There is no doubt that prolonged pain can erode self-esteem and confidence if doctors fail to help, friends look the other way, and the future seems bleak and lonely. If chronic pain were simply a repetition of acute pains, this would not happen. But in that case, we should be unable to relieve chronic pain by providing care and comfort.

6

The Unanswered Cry

In March 1988, the National Health Service (NHS) ombudsman reported on an incident at the modern, prestigious Royal Free Hospital in North London. The ombudsman (the word is borrowed from a traditional Danish post) has the duty of investigating complaints; he is paid from public funds, but is independent of NHS authorities and government departments.

The allegation concerned an 85-year-old woman, Mrs. Dorothea Mangold, who had been admitted to the hospital with a fractured thigh after a fall at home. At 2 AM one night, she was in such severe pain that she called for help. The response by the (male) charge nurse in the ward was to wheel her to a dark room. Mrs. Mangold's son, citing his mother's account, told the ombudsman: "There was no bell, no light switch, and no other human being in the room and she was just dumped there. . . . She lay there begging for help in the darkness, the pain becoming worse in her leg, while the emphysema began to afflict her following the emotional shock of what had happened. She was left there, she thinks, for about 4 to 6 hours."

The ombudsman found that this was a true account, and he commented: "The need to move Mrs. Mangold to the treatment room and her consequent distress might have been avoided had she been treated in a more sensitive manner." He also criticized the hospital authorities for their response to Mr.

Mangold's letters of complaint; they replied defending the charge nurse's action and denying that any mistakes had been made. Tom Mangold is a television reporter with the BBC, experienced in pursuing inquiries and detecting coverups. Most people don't know that there is such a person as the NHS ombudsman. For that matter, not all hospital patients have relatives who visit them, care about their welfare, and make a fuss if they are badly treated.

How could such a shocking incident have occurred? True, it is difficult to keep up a satisfactory standard of patient care in Britain's understaffed and underfunded hospitals. But if we reflect more deeply, we can see that Mrs. Mangold was the victim of an attitude toward pain that, despite the fresh thinking of recent years, is still far too prevalent. If put into words (which it seldom is), the attitude would be "We can't do anything about pain and anyway it's not our job, so we don't want to think about it." Indeed, shutting the sufferer from pain in a dark room without a call bell is an eloquent symbol of this attitude.

No one has counted how many cries for help—in hospitals or in homes—go unanswered. No one could count how many cries are stifled and never uttered. The reasons for the neglect of pain are varied and quite complicated, but it is important to examine them.

DOCTOR AND PATIENT

Few relationships are more delicate or more complex than the relationship between doctor and patient. The patient listens to the doctor's every word, and even scrutinizes facial expressions, to pick up clues. The doctor tries to avoid saying or doing anything that may alarm the patient needlessly or exacerbate a medical condition. The poet and cleric John Donne, writing at a time when he was himself a sick man, described the situation with sensitive insight:

> I observe the Physician, with the same diligence, as he the disease; I see he fears, and I fear with him. . . . I fear the more, because he disguises his fear, and I see it with the more sharpness, because he would not have me see it. He knows that his fear shall not disorder the practice and exercise of his Art, but he knows that my fear may disorder the effect and working of his practice. As the ill affections of the spleen complicate and mingle themselves with every infirmity of the body, so doth fear insinuate itself in every action or passion of the mind.

In this situation, the doctor is tempted to distance himself from the patient and prevent the transmission (either way) of emotions such as fear and anxiety. If only the patient were a piece of machinery, incapable of feeling, suffering, speaking, or weeping, if only the doctor could go to work like a repairman working on a defective plumbing system, how much easier the doctor's life would be! Indeed, doctors have behaved for generations, and many of them still behave, as though this were the case. The assumption is that, when the bodily organism is not functioning properly, it is the doctor, not the patient, who knows what is wrong. Even to explain to the patient is an act of grace on the doctor's part. (This attitude is strengthened by the disparities in social class, status, and education that often separate doctor and patient.) The feelings of the patient are not the doctor's concern; distress and suffering are to be dealt with by the nursing staff if the patient is in hospital, or by family and friends if the patient is at home. And pain is very much a matter of how the patient is feeling—a subjective experience, as we have defined it. On these assumptions, there is a logic in excluding pain from the medical sphere.

It was natural that such attitudes should become dominant in the nineteenth century because the sciences were imbued with a mechanistic brand of materialism. Our planet was seen as a machine, powered by the sun to produce the means of life. The human body was a machine, powered by a pump called the heart. Irregular heartbeat and hardening of the arteries were signs of malfunction, just as a spluttering carburetor is a sign of malfunction in a car. Pain was an irrelevance and a distraction—or, at most, one symptom among others. It was never seen as an experience of the whole person, to be understood in terms broader than the symptomatic.

In 1894, a philosopher and psychologist named H. R. Marshall put forward the theory that pain is not a sensory event, but a quality that may attach to any sensory event. For instance, he suggested, hearing music played out of tune is painful for a musician. In the heyday of materialism, he was laughed at by most medical authorities. But we can now see that his theory was immensely fruitful. He was making a unity of sensation and perception, divided since the time of Descartes.

Inevitably, a conservative medical hierarchy saw no reason why doctors should study or think about pain as a problem in its own right. That conservative hierarchy still controls medical education in most countries. In 1988, two researchers at Southampton University looked at the training provided in Britain's 28 medical schools (34). They found that four of these schools offered no teaching whatever related to pain and pain control, and the others offered an average of three and a half *hours* in a 5-year course. Only 10 of the schools included questions on pain control in examinations. Only six offered the students experience in a pain clinic. The researchers also examined all 250 postgraduate courses advertised in recent issues of the *Lancet* and the *British Medical Journal*. Only one had any bearing on pain control, and it was aimed at doctors already specializing in the field.

To find out what doctors actually do, the researchers sent a questionnaire to all general practitioners in an area surrounding a large hospital that has a pain clinic. At the time of this research, pain clinics—the first of which was instituted in Tacoma by J. J. Bonica in 1947—were well established and to be found in many hospitals in Britain as well as in the United States. They will receive fuller description later, but their basic function is to bring together a multidisciplinary team to deal specifically with pain conditions.

The replies to the questionnaire showed that all the doctors were aware of the clinic's existence, but they were in no hurry to direct patients there. The average time lapse between a complaint of pain and referral to the clinic was over 5 years. Presumably, the clinic was regarded as a last resort, or a way of passing on a troublesome patient. While 87% of the doctors knew that the clinic could treat cancer pain, comparable scores were 34% with regard to pain from osteoarthritis, 22% for migraine, and 14% for tension headaches. Very few (less than 2%) of the referrals were for migraine or tension headache, although the clinic was particularly well equipped to treat these types of pain.

THE WARNING SIGNAL

There is another reason why doctors have been, and to some extent still are, reluctant to treat pain as an enemy. This was a belief in the positive usefulness of pain. It is pain—so it was thought—that gives the first warning of a serious disease, such as cancer. Doctors, therefore, felt justified in being extremely sparing in the use of pain-killing drugs; to suppress pain, it was argued, was to suppress useful evidence. The whole theory stemmed from a philosophy that everything in life was there for a purpose (whether ordained by God, by Nature, by the life force, or whatever). For those who accepted that principle, a purpose had to be found for pain too.

It is certainly true, and indeed obvious, that sudden, acute pain serves a purpose. If an injury to your hand causes pain, you very quickly remove it from the electrified wire or the cutting edge of the saw. If there were no pain to bring about this reaction—as in the rare case of Miss C.—we should incur much graver injuries. It is also true, as we recall from memories of childhood, that experience of pain teaches us how to avoid it on future occasions. The proverb "A burnt child fears the fire" is founded on accurate observation. However, it by no means follows that what is true of acute pain caused by external injury is equally true of chronic pain, arising from internal causes or from no ascertainable cause. Once again, we must take into account the historical context in which beliefs are shaped. In past centuries there was just as much acute pain as there is now—there have always been fires, accidents, and war wounds—but long-lasting chronic pain was less familiar.

In 1939, this belief in the value of pain was bluntly challenged by René Leriche, a distinguished surgeon, who wrote:

> Physicians too readily claim that pain is a reaction of the risks of disease. . . . Reaction of defense? Against whom? Against what? Against the cancer which not infrequently gives little trouble until quite late? Against heart afflictions, which always develop quietly? . . . One must reject, then, this false conception of beneficent pain.

Leriche was right, and accumulating knowledge since 1939 has only proved how right he was. We have already mentioned silent heart attacks—that is, attacks that are unaccompanied by pain and therefore have no warning signal. Millions of people who present themselves for examination, whether as a prudent checkup or to take out an insurance policy, prove to have an inadequate blood supply to the heart, carrying the risk of a heart attack, but have never experienced any pain. The pain comes after the heart attack, not before.

We have also explained that cancer is generally painless in the early stage of development, and sometimes painless in quite a late stage, or even up to the moment of death. The pain that goes with cancer—which can, alas, be excruciating—is not generated by the growth in the lung or the stomach, but by secondary effects, by the pressure of cancerous tissue on nerves, or by the spreading of the cancer to other structures, such as bones. These events occur when the cancer is advanced, and when a cure is difficult or impossible. A lung cancer can grow to the size of a grapefruit without being noticed. A brain tumor can progress to serious, even lethal, proportions before it causes headaches—and, when it does, they can easily be mistaken for ordinary tension headaches.

The case of the British writer John Morgan is sad but instructive. When he was making a routine visit to the dentist, and experiencing no pain of any kind, the dentist observed something suspicious and said, "I think you should see your doctor." Morgan had cancer of the mouth. He was thankful that it had been detected early, but it was not early enough. The cancer proved to be ineradicable, and he died within 2 years after suffering severe pain in the final months of his life. The pain had failed to make its appearance when it might have been useful.

We could go on. The pain that accompanies arthritis is not a warning signal, because weakening of the joints has already set in. Postoperative pain is plainly not a warning signal; it comes after the operation. It is equally obvious that phantom limb pain, persisting for years after an amputation, cannot warn of anything. In all these cases, pain has no point and no value. It is simply our enemy.

IT'S ALL IN THE HEAD

Another justification for the neglect of pain is the idea—sometimes spelled out, sometimes implicit—that pain is somehow optional. According to this line of thinking, which gives rise to common phrases such as "it's all in the head," there are people who give in to pain and people who don't. Those who do are weak or cowardly or, at best, ignorant of ways of rising above the assault of pain. These people deserve neither our respect nor our sympathy.

Our dominant tradition teaches us to admire those who bear pain without flinching, from the Spartan boy who never uttered a cry while the fox was chewing his arm, all the way to James Bond and Rambo. Characters who keep their heads down and avoid trouble—Schweik, Gunner Asch, or Jack Boyle in *Juno and the Paycock*—evoke our amusement but not our admiration. Stoicism in the face of pain is a test of manhood; it is also cited, sometimes, to show that women are braver than men. The Masai in Kenya and Tanzania arrange the social rank of men by their ability to show no reaction to progressively more severe injury. Infliction of pain as an initiation rite is supposed to be a custom observed only by anthropologists in places like New Guinea, but—as recent courts-martial have revealed—it happens in the British Army too. Authors of British upper-class autobiographies proudly record the canings and the exercise to exhaustion point in their schools, which shaped them (in their own estimation) into splendid characters. Their counterparts in German universities took pride in dueling scars until well into the twentieth century. Today, young people in aerobic classes work enthusiastically to pass the pain barrier.

The most insidious effect of this strand in our culture is to make people who are in genuine pain feel guilty. If "it's all in the head," why must they feel so miserable? Is it really their own fault? A question commonly encountered by experts on pain is whether there are people with high pain thresholds. The very frequency of this question reveals anxiety. Those who feel pain badly (have a low threshold) are seeking permission to complain and reassurance that they are not morally to blame. Those who can claim to have a high threshold are entitled to feel superior to their less fortunate brethren.

Distinctions between those who are sensitive to pain and those who are not can be individual, but can also be made to apply to entire ethnic groups or nationalities. We have noted the belief that women of "primitive races" don't feel the pain of childbirth as white women do. Such notions are also quite consoling for the man in uniform beating up someone with whom he does not identify, be it in Belfast or in Gaza.

THE MORAL VALUE MYTH

But of all the myths that bar the way to the relief of pain, the most potent and persistent is its alleged moral value. This belief pervades the whole of our Western culture and is deeply rooted in—as well as legitimized by—our dominant religion, Christianity. Among the great world religions, Christianity is the only one whose founder perished in circumstances of apparent defeat and humiliation, instead of rounding off triumphant conquests, like Mohammed, or gaining a satisfying acceptance as a respected teacher, like Buddha. Not only this, but Jesus Christ was doomed to an agonizing death through crucifixion, a form of execution that had been specially designed to be intensely painful. For 2000 years, Christians have lived with the infinitely multiplied vision of Christ on the cross, reproduced in thousands of paintings and statues, over the altars of churches, and on the crucifix worn round the neck. It cannot fail to generate profound feelings of reverence, in which the concept of Christ as redeemer and the concept of Christ as a sufferer are merged.

Christian teaching stresses that this suffering was knowingly and voluntarily accepted by Christ. His example was followed, during the next three centuries when Christianity was a persecuted religion, by saints and martyrs who refused to save their lives by renouncing their faith and also went voluntarily to cruel and painful deaths—savaged by lions, broken on the wheel, and so forth. (Some of the stories of martyrdom are mythical, but that makes no difference in their effectiveness.) They too are immortalized in ubiquitous works of art and have become the objects of worship and the recipients of prayer.

A later aspect of Christian history is even more extraordinary. Long after Christianity had become a dominant (and indeed a persecuting) religion, long after martyrdom had become unnecessary, devout Christians by the score inflicted pain and suffering *on themselves* in order to raise their moral stature. Some of their techniques were as ingenious as they were horrifying. The Blessed Henry Suso, a German who lived in the fourteenth century, left a book-length account of the torments he devised over a period of 20 years (he eventually decided that he had done enough). A brief extract will suffice:

He secretly caused an undergarment to be made for him; and in the undergarment he had strips of leather fixed, into which a hundred and fifty brass nails, pointed and filed sharp, were driven, and the points of the nails were always turned toward the flesh. He had this garment made very tight, and so arranged as to go round him and fasten in front, in order that it might fit the closer to his body and the pointed nails might be driven into his flesh.

The kind of thinking that motivated his behavior is very frankly and clearly indicated in an adulatory biography of Saint Marguerite Marie Alacoque, founder of the cult of the Sacred Heart:

Her love of pain and suffering was insatiable. . . . She said that she could cheerfully live till the day of judgement, provided she might always have matter for suffering for God, but that to live a single day without suffering would be intolerable. She said again that she was devoured with two unassuageable fevers, one for the Holy Communion, the other for suffering, humiliation, and annihilation. "Nothing but pain," she continually said in her letters, "makes my life supportable."

It is worth noting that Marguerite Marie did not live in the remote Middle Ages, but from 1647 to 1690; that the cult of the Sacred Heart reached its apogee in the nineteenth century, when the great Basilica that towers over Paris was built; that the biography we have quoted was published in 1894; and that Marguerite Marie was canonized as recently as 1920.

Indeed, belief in the necessity and desirability of pain is still flourishing today and is recommended by the highest religious authorities. In 1984, Pope John Paul II delivered a pronouncement "in liturgical remembrance of the Blessed Mary, Virgin of Lourdes." Quoting a sentence in one of the epistles of St. Paul—"I am now happy in the suffering that I endure for you"—the Pope explained:

The joy comes from the discovery of the meaning of suffering, and such a discovery, even if Paul of Tarsus writes these words in a deeply personal way, is at the same time valid for others.

He went on to expand the point thus:

What we express with the word "suffering" seems to be particularly *essential to the nature of Man*. [The Pope's italics.] . . . Suffering seems to belong to Man's transcendence; it is one of those points at which Man is in a certain way "destined" to overcome himself, and is mysteriously presented as such.

A later passage reads:

Sharing in the sufferings of Christ is, at the same time, suffering for the Kingdom of God. In the just eyes of God, before His justice, those who share in Christ's sufferings become worthy of this Kingdom. Through their sufferings they, in a sense, pay back the boundless price of our redemption.

And the Pope concluded: "Suffering contains, as it were, an appeal to Man's moral greatness and spiritual maturity."

Such a view is not confined to the Catholic Church. The writer C. S. Lewis, a member of the (Protestant) Church of England, devoted a short book to what he called "the problem of pain" and told his readers:

Christianity . . . is not a system into which we have to fit the awkward fact of pain. . . . In a sense, it creates, rather than solves, the problem of pain, for pain would be no problem unless, side by side with our daily experience of this painful world, we had received what we think is a good assurance that ultimate reality is righteous and loving.

Not surprisingly, the advice that Lewis offered was "When pain is to be borne, a little courage helps more than much knowledge."

Not all Christians, it is fair to say, would accept the doctrines thus enunciated. Many of them, no doubt—along with agnostics or followers of other religions—are simply appalled by pain when they encounter it and fail to see that it has any benefits. Still, Europeans and Americans in general inherit the cultural and intellectual influence exerted across the centuries by Christianity. The idea of suffering as an "appeal to moral greatness" inevitably colors the outlook of millions of ordinary people, of writers and artists, of teachers and educators—and of doctors too. C. S. Lewis was able to add to his book a contribution by a doctor, who wrote:

> Long–continued pain . . . is often accepted with little or no complaint and great strength and resignation are developed. Pride is humbled or, at times, results in a determination to conceal suffering. . . . Pain provides an opportunity for heroism; the opportunity is seized with surprising frequency.

We are influenced, too, by the literature on which we have been brought up. The great novels of the nineteenth century repeatedly depict stricken and dying men, women, and children whose characters are ennobled and refined by suffering, and who exhibit virtues that were beyond their reach when they were healthy. Thus, we are led to admire—in real life as well as in fiction—people who endure pain with calm, uncomplaining resignation. This behavior earns particular approval in hospitals, especially when coupled with consideration for other patients and for the hospital staff. It's no wonder that Mrs. Mangold was punished for failing to live up to the ideal.

All the same, the myth is a distortion of reality. Far from being ennobling, pain is a demeaning experience. Even moderate pain, preventing the victim from living a normal life, can be humiliating. Severe pain, reducing a human being to an unrecognizable, writhing, screaming creature, is intensely humiliating. The true morality is not to seek value in it, but to detest it and combat it.

But the myth is comforting for those of us—the majority—who are not in pain. As La Rochefoucauld put it: "We all have enough strength to bear the misfortunes of others."

7

Pain Behavior

We have already stated that pain is an experience a human being undergoes, not simply as a structure of body tissue and nerves, but as an individual person. It is impossible for one person to share another's pain, or to know exactly what the other person is feeling, even with the closest links of affection and sympathy. We also stated as a corollary that pain cannot be measured. To be strictly accurate, it cannot even be observed. When a doctor examines a patient in the terminal stage of cancer, he may deduce from all kinds of symptoms that the patient is in severe pain, but he is observing the symptoms, not the pain itself.

Pain behavior, however, can be observed with a high degree of accuracy, and in some respects can be measured. By pain behavior, we mean everything a person does when in pain and every change of state he exhibits. There are several varieties of pain behavior—or, to adopt another terminology, several kinds of response to pain.

One distinct class consists of involuntary responses, which a person does not consciously initiate and cannot prevent. These include changes in heart rate, brain activity, blood pressure, gastric activity, sweating, and muscle tension. They can be measured with precision by such instruments as the electroencelograph. Although these responses normally appear when expected, they can be affected by individual personality, past experiences, or cultural background, so they are not automatic in the sense of being inevitable and invariable. This is why we are justified in regarding them as a form of behavior. But, since they are not employed as a means of communication, they tell us relatively little about the distress and suffering that are the essence of pain itself.

Next, we have a class of responses such as wincing, twisting and writhing, clutching the place where pain is felt, groaning, and weeping. Distorted facial expressions, noted by many artists as indicative of pain, also fall into this category. This behavior is on the borderline between the voluntary and the involuntary. Some people who engage in this kind of pain behavior—notably children, of course—feel that they are unable to help it. Some could refrain from it with an effort, but feel they have a right to it and use it (consciously or otherwise) to attract attention and sympathy. Some, however, regard this pain behavior as shameful and succeed, partly or even completely, in checking it. With the pain behavior we are now considering, individual personality and cultural background are definitely relevant.

An important place in pain behavior belongs to verbal responses. The use of language is, of course, the ability that outstandingly distinguishes human beings from other animals and is a resource on which people in pain are very likely to draw. We see how valuable it is when we try to establish the nature and location of pain in a baby without language, or in a pet dog or cat. Doctors use spoken (or, even better, written) descriptions of pain as an aid in diagnosis, and then in charting the progress of an illness. So far as we are able to penetrate the mystery of pain itself, we are indebted to the words of articulate sufferers.

However, a caution is necessary. Talking about pain is, obviously, conscious and fully voluntary, and individuals will therefore vary extensively in what they say, even if they are trying to report their experience objectively. Not surprisingly, some people exaggerate their pain in a bid for sympathy and help. A patient in a busy, understaffed hospital ward can scarcely be blamed for employing that strategy. Others, on the other hand, seek to gain credit, or achieve a sense of pride, by denying or at least minimizing real pain. ("It's all right, doctor, it's nothing much.") The French diplomat Charles-Maurice de Talleyrand remarked, "Speech is given to man to disguise his thoughts." We can sometimes paraphrase this as "to disguise his pain."

In connection with verbal complaints of pain (and in this context we can include screaming and weeping), cultural background and social standards are highly significant. An interesting book, based on observations in a New York hospital for veterans, describes the pain behavior of men of various ethnic origins (76). It was found that men of long-standing American descent reply to questioning by describing their pain as bearable, Irishmen withdraw into silence, while Jews and Italians feel no inhibition about complaining loudly.

Studies have been made with the aim of establishing a relationship between pain expression (in speech or by screaming) and pain tolerance (the ability to endure pain without finding it unbearable and demanding relief). The conclusion from these studies is that to correlate pain expression with pain perception is an error. In one study, it was found that introverted, neurotic people had a low tolerance of pain. However, it was just these people who, because they were given to silent brooding, refrained from pain expression.

BEHAVIOR IN CHRONIC PAIN

Consideration of pain behavior is most significant in relation to long-lasting chronic pain, rather than to sudden acute pain. If a person is stung by a hornet, that person's behavior (voluntary and involuntary) will be fairly predictable whether he or she is an American university professor, a French artist, or a Chinese tea picker. In any case, the behavior doesn't matter much because both the pain and the injury will be of brief duration, and recovery will not be significantly aided or hindered by this behavior. But when a person is likely to be in pain for years—for example, in cases of osteoarthritis—the situation is far more serious. What is needed then is an ability to live with pain: that is, to evolve and maintain patterns of behavior that prevent pain from totally dominating life. A person who succeeds in this will be raising the level of pain tolerance.

We sometimes meet a person in chronic pain whose character and behavior seem the same as before the pain began, so that friends say, "You'd never guess if you didn't know." More often, however, we find that chronic pain has altered a personality—perhaps for the better, perhaps for the worse. One person may have discovered hitherto-unsuspected resources of inner strength and courage; another may simply have become miserable and embittered. The ways in which individuals reveal these characteristics are their patterns of pain behavior. But, as well as being revealed, the characteristics are also progressively reinforced.

One of the saddest aspects of the pain experience is that, at the time when a person needs to be serene, mature, and capable of confronting difficulties, pain is tending to make him anxious and helpless. Pain is humiliating because one needs assistance in doing things one had taken for granted—dressing and undressing, getting in and out of the bathtub, going upstairs, going for a walk. While the normal person does not mind being alone (and may enjoy periods of solitude), the person in chronic pain is compelled to fear being alone. Anxiety is constant because the pain may unpredictably become worse at any time of the day or night.

Instead of the independence and control associated with adult life, one is thrown back into the dependence and insecurity of childhood. Loss of employment and being forced to stay at home all day emphasize this state of affairs. In this enforced regression to childhood, it is difficult not to feel—as a child would—that the pain is a punishment. Readers will remember that we have pointed out the historic association between pain and punishment, through the dual meaning of the word *peine*.

The childhood situation is likely to produce child-like behavior. In his book *Pain: A Psychophysiological Analysis* (60), Richard Sternbach writes:

> We ask what we have done to deserve such pain, and think back to make a connection between some action of ours and the onset of the pain. We implore others to help us, to take away the hurt. . . . We beg for forgiveness, we say we are sorry. . . . We act as though we are dealing with a parental figure who will harm us if we are bad, if we do or have done bad things, or even have bad thoughts. As contriteness fails, we throw ourselves on the mercy of, not the forgiving parent, but the compassionate one, the helpful one, the one who would kiss the hurt away if we asked for help.

Sternbach goes on to remark that such child-like hopes and wishes are discernible in what people say when in pain. Stressing the awfulness of the pain is a straightforward cry for help. But the person who voices no complaint and does *not* demand help is staking a claim to parental approval for "not being a cry-baby," for being "a brave little man."

GUILT, ANXIETY, AND DEPRESSION

The concept of pain as punishment tends to generate feelings of guilt, or to intensify them if they already exist. There may, indeed, be objective reasons for a consciousness of guilt. A person may have invited an accident through recklessness or negligence. He may, through belligerence and a tendency to violence, have got into a fight and sustained an injury that causes chronic pain. He may have good cause to ascribe his cancer or his angina pectoris to years of heavy smoking or unwise eating. In the majority of cases, however, the guilt is imaginary. People who have led scrupulously careful lives and even avoided undue stress do, unfortunately, fall victim to cancer or have heart attacks. We have noted that back pain—the most common kind of chronic pain—typically appears for no ascertainable reason. But the presence of a guilt feeling is not necessarily related to its rationality.

Whether justified by objective facts or not, guilt is a useless response to pain, because it obviously fails to make the pain go away or even diminish. Worse than useless, it can well be harmful. The person who allows his mind to dwell obsessively on guilt is, in effect, seeking to punish himself, and the most direct way of punishing himself is to feel more pain. Intense feelings of guilt are likely to reduce the level of pain tolerance.

Moreover, if admitting one's guilt and saying "I'm sorry" does no good—if forgiveness and compassion are not forthcoming—then it seems to follow that the guilt was even graver than it was thought to be. Thus, a vicious circle is set up. Confession of guilt leads to yet more obsessive brooding on guilt, and to sharper anxiety. Someone who is caught in this trap has little chance of learning to live with pain.

When anxiety is severe and unrelieved, the outcome is likely to be depression. In everyday speech, the word "depression" is used quite loosely. If someone says, "I feel terribly depressed today," nothing very alarming is implied. Scientifically, however, depression is a precise, definable term for a form of mental illness. Psychiatrists use the term "major depression" to mean a depression unjustified by any objective source. Such a major depression needs to be treated as a problem in its own right. Clearly, a person who is suffering from both pain and depression is in heavy trouble.

In this predicament, daily life become unendurable. It appears that the only escape from the dual misery of pain and depression is to dull the mind. The obvious way to do this is to demand stronger, more frequent doses of drugs prescribed for pain, such as morphine. We shall discuss the use of these drugs in detail later; here, we can say briefly that it is right to use them generously for the relief of pain, and that the danger of addiction has been much exaggerated. However, the proper use of morphine is not to provide an escape from reality but, on the contrary, to alleviate pain so that real life can be managed more successfully. When depression is the motive for requiring a drug, the possibility of addiction does come into serious consideration.

There is another drug that effectively dulls the mind and can be obtained legally without a medical prescription—namely, alcohol. Because a glass of brandy is a normal, socially accepted way of relieving pain (for instance, after a hard session with the dentist), regular use of alcohol is a temptation for people in chronic pain, and it is all too easy for regular use to become excessive and addictive. An experience of pain has been the point of departure for a large number of alcoholics.

Finally, the feeling that life is unendurable can lead to a conviction that it must be terminated: in other words, to suicide. A great deal can be said, and has been said, about the ethics of suicide and about the related question of euthanasia. Our own view is that when suicide is decided on to resolve a hopeless situation—especially in the case of a person in great pain, with no prospect of regaining good health—it can be a rational choice, manifesting a dignity and courage worthy of respect. But when the impulse toward suicide arises from the condition of depression, which could probably have been treated in one way or another, then a life is being lost unnecessarily. The sad fact is that thousands of lives every year are destroyed in this tragic way.

THE PATTERN OF SELF-PITY

Among the patterns of pain behavior (the variety is larger than we can cover here), probably the most common is self-pity.

It is highly verbalized; the self-pitying person is much given to elaborate descriptions of pain, supplemented by running commentaries and heightened at times by moaning, groaning, or sobbing. It is distinct from depression, in that the person suffering from depression tends to be silent and uncommunicative.

Self-pity in those with poor health or classified as "delicate" was an accepted behavior pattern in the nineteenth century—especially (it seems) in England, especially in the leisured classes, and especially for women, whose husbands could gain applause by showing consideration for them. Today, we are more inclined to regard self-pity as an unattractive or even irritating emotion, and to condemn people for yielding to it. This kind of disapproval is resented by the self-pitier, understandably enough. Pain is real, and anyone in pain is tempted to say, "Don't I have a right to feel sorry for myself?" The attitude that self-pity is justified and "natural" is, of course, the reason why it is so common. In fact, a certain amount of open recognition of pain—a certain amount of grumbling or cursing or whatever comes naturally—can be therapeutic, and total denial of pain is seldom healthy. The point at which we should become suspicious of self-pity is when it develops into a continual, unbroken concentration on one's own misfortunes—when, in Thornton Wilder's vivid phrase, someone "listens to his body as if it were a Stradivarius."

This gives us a clue to a feature of self-pity that is not always recognized and is unlikely to be admitted by the person who manifests it. Self-pity soon becomes, if it was not at the outset, an indulgence that supplies a form of pleasure. Unhappiness as well as happiness can be pursued, cultivated, and elaborated. Misery can be a way of life.

As the word implies, self-pity is an essentially selfish stance. The sufferer feels free to make incessant complaints and demands, and to require that life should revolve around him (or her, as the case may be). The house must be quiet, he must never be left alone, someone must always be within call and prepared to drop other activities. He enjoys the privilege of being short-tempered and speaking sharply, but if anyone else behaves similarly it is proof of heartless cruelty.

This behavior has a purpose, conscious or otherwise: it is manipulative and exploitative. Pain is being used strategically, just as, in other situations, charm or beauty can be used. It is a weapon wielded to gain power. Although this type of person represents himself as powerless, and may indeed believe himself to be powerless, he is making himself the most powerful figure in his environment. Were he to be deprived of pain, he would be deprived of this source of power. Thus, when the pain is actually relieved by a new kind of treatment or an appropriate drug, he accepts the improvement grudgingly rather than gratefully and clings to his familiar behavior pattern. The habits of self-pity, of complaining and demanding, cannot be abandoned without a positive effort which he is reluctant to make.

Sooner or later, there is a price to be paid for self-pity. It is generally paid by others in the pain sufferer's family or environment, but it may well be paid by the pain sufferer himself. As others come to feel that they are being sacrificed to his demands, he alienates the affection and sympathy that he seeks. There are rebellions and conflicts. He launches accusations: "You don't love me! You don't care about me! You wish I was dead!" The person who is the target of these accusations denies them, but feels miserably that there is some truth in them. Eventually the situation becomes untenable, and the relationship (or marriage) collapses under the excessive strain placed on it. This leaves the sufferer with increased grounds for self-pity, but with some consolation from this proof that he has been badly treated and abandoned. Perhaps he now enters an institution. This cannot solve his problem; he is unlikely to be popular with the other residents, or with the staff. As a strategy to secure power and satisfaction, self-pity has proved to be remarkably counterproductive. Even if events do not develop as in this scenario, it is not a behavior pattern that can contribute toward a successful adaptation.

THE PATTERN OF DEFIANCE

Another behavior pattern appears, superficially, to be the direct opposite of the self-pitying pattern (although the two have some features in common, notably the desire to be the center of attention). We can call this the pattern of defiance. The person who selects it announces that he refuses to accept his pain—he intends to fight it. His dominant emotion is resentment, amounting to anger. The real target of the anger is the pain, but it is directed against other people: perhaps against those believed to have caused the pain (if it was an injury), perhaps against family members who are deemed insufficiently helpful, but particularly against doctors. This person insists that there must be a surefire way of removing his pain, and failure to achieve this must be ascribed to the incompetence or indifference of the medical profession.

Therefore, he throws himself enthusiastically into the activity known in medical circles as doctor shopping. When one doctor fails to give satisfaction, he turns to another. At the hospital, he makes the round of the specialist clinics. If he decides that a doctor has given him the wrong treatment, he complains to his Member of Parliament (in Britain) or brings a lawsuit for malpractice (in the United States). Losing faith in the orthodox medical profession, he goes on to practitioners of alternative medicine. He may indeed get genuine help from them, but he may end up as a customer for quacks and charlatans.

Many doctor shoppers are sufferers from back pain, because this kind of pain can be regarded by the layman as a straightforward mechanical malfunctioning to be "fixed" by a repair job. The doctor shopper therefore demands surgery, and if he is shopping on the private market and his purse is capacious enough, he gets surgery. Some back patients in America have had six or more operations and are ready for more.

Typically, the person who adopts the behavior of defiance rejects any suggestion that there could be a psychological component of his pain. If he is advised to consult a psychiatrist, his anger quickly flares. The insinuation, as he sees it, is that his pain is imaginary—that it is a delusion. "Are you telling me it's all in the mind?" he demands. He fails to appreciate that pain, while perfectly real, is both in the mind and in the body, being a unitary experience of the whole person; thus, to bring in the psychiatrist is simply to attack it from another angle. Even if he agrees to a session with a psychiatrist, he goes into the interview in a suspicious spirit and probably derives little benefit from it—which, of course, confirms his hostility.

We should not too easily deride the person who adopts the pattern of defiance. When someone is in pain, it is quite reasonable for him to explore every possibility of relief. The authors of this book are not dogmatic defenders of the medical profession; there certainly are doctors who are lazy or careless, who make errors in diagnosis and treatment, and whose stock of knowledge is not kept up to date. It can credibly be argued that doctor shoppers are performing a service for the rest of us by keeping doctors up to the mark.

When all this is conceded, however, the pattern of defiance is in most cases an inappropriate and unproductive response to pain. These are the cases of chronic pain in which, regrettably, there really is no known technique for getting rid of the pain. The sufferer has to be advised to find ways of living with the pain and controlling it, which inevitably means that he cannot live as he did when in perfect health. The defier reacts to this advice with the charge that the doctor is evading his responsibility, his duty to cure. But it is really the defier who is evading a responsibility and shielding himself from reality. Every pain sufferer is in need of help, including professional help, but he also needs to muster his own resources. Only thus can he hope to keep the pain within bounds and prevent it from ruling his life.

THE PATTERN OF RESIGNATION

Yet another possible behavior pattern is complete resignation to pain. The person who adopts this pattern invariably gives up his job when chronic pain sets in, even if the pain is not severe enough to make this absolutely necessary. If offered an option of working part time or working from home, he rejects it. Any proposed interest or hobby—learning a language, taking correspondence courses, or whatever—is also rejected as beyond his capacity. He ceases to see friends and declines the offer of visits on the grounds that he would be unable to keep up a conversation. This behavior is not exactly the cultivation of unhappiness, but it is certainly the cultivation of helplessness.

Unlike the complaining, demanding person we have described, this person chooses to suffer in silence (or perhaps with a just perceptible sigh). Rather than insisting on sympathy, he ignores it when it is expressed. If someone asks whether he has any needs or wishes, he replies, "No, thank you—just leave me alone."

This behavior amounts to, and can be explained as, a willing acceptance of punishment. The deliberately chosen solitude imitates the loneliness of the child who, for some offense, has been excluded from the family circle, or sent up to a bedroom. (The self-isolating person often prefers a darkened room with drawn curtains.) The form of punishment he imagines is rejection, abandonment. But instead of protesting against this punishment and complaining that it is unfair, he welcomes and perpetuates it. There is nothing like pain for reinforcing a latent tendency to masochism.

The pattern of resignation is tempting because it can be presented as courageous, dignified, and honest, or at least sensible and realistic. But although it may be more realistic than defiance, it is not entirely realistic. It is never true that there is nothing to be done about pain. As we have said repeatedly, one can work out a way of living with and controlling the pain—or one can fail to do so. To choose a pattern of resignation is to choose a way of life that has no place for anything but pain, and this must necessarily exacerbate the experience of suffering.

It will be evident by now that the patterns we have discussed are all, in quite different ways, negative approaches to the problem that pain presents. A positive approach is always possible. It involves a willingness to grapple with the pain and to assume a personal responsibility for the required effort.

We have concentrated in this chapter on the choices open to the person in pain. Fortunately, a great deal can be done *for* this person. The content of the next three chapters is the treatment of pain.

8

Treatment of Pain with Medicine

A key concept of modern Chinese medicine is "We recruit the patient to be a member of his own treatment team." If implemented in a Western society, that crucial step would require a change of attitude by both therapist and patient. The doctor would have to relinquish his authoritarian status as priest–healer. The patient would have to step up his activity and involvement and work hard to improve his knowledge and understanding. In most hospitals today, the patient's admission is a rite of passage whereby he sacrifices his independent identity. Stripped of his familiar clothes, dressed in a bizarre smock, wearing a numbered identity tag on his wrist like a newborn baby, he reverts to an infantile status, with food, shelter, and activity all regulated by omnipotent adults. Just as "Daddy knows best" for the child, "Doctor knows best" for the patient.

True, in an important sense the doctor does know best; every competent physician is a living storehouse of knowledge, skill, and experience. Considerations of time, status, and efficiency persuade the patient to be quiet and let the experts get on with the job. In a repair workshop, assuming that the customer trusts the mechanic and knows nothing about motor engines, this is doubtless a good idea. But an ailing patient is not a damaged engine, and his cooperation and activity will aid his recovery. Our aim in this chapter is to provide resources for that cooperation by describing the nature and effect of various forms of treatment. We begin by explaining certain key words that we shall be using frequently.

CAUSE AND EFFECT

The phrase *post hoc ergo propter hoc* ("after that, therefore because of that") was recognized by thinkers in ancient Rome as a confusing fallacy. In the treatment of pain, this must constantly be kept in mind. Few painful conditions are stable. Pains such as headaches, backaches, and neuromuscular disorders may rise to a climax followed by a spontaneous remission, or unexplained period of relief. If a doctor is lucky enough to appear at the right moment, the remission can be attributed to his effective therapy. Unfortunately, deterioration can also be a feature of many painful conditions. The doctor is then the target of anger, alienation, and accusations of incompetence.

In past centuries, when medicine was more of an art than a science, it often happened that a doctor, aware of his inability to do anything useful for a patient, prescribed a so-called medicine that was actually an innocuous concoction of sugar and water. Swallowing the stuff would at least make the patient feel that the doctor cared, and the doctor (speaking in Latin, of course) may well have murmured to himself, "*Placebo*" ("I will please"). The word *placebo* eventually became a noun, defined in the Oxford Dictionary as "a medicine given more to please than to benefit the patient."

Then doctors in hospitals began to make a surprising observation: the placebos did seem to do the patients some good. They experienced relief from pain, and in some cases their medical condition improved or they actually achieved an unexpected cure. Studies were made: first blind studies (the patient did not know whether he was getting his usual medicine or a placebo) and then double-blind (the doctor was also prevented from knowing which he was administering). In a study of people with postoperative pain, 75% reported relief from a strong dose of morphine, but 35% of another group reported relief from a placebo. Clearly, the percentage who would report relief if left alone and given nothing would be practically zero. Similarly, in a study of cancer patients who responded satisfactorily to morphine, a high percentage responded just as well to a placebo. But if the placebo was repeated, the benefit faded and relief from pain resulted only from real morphine.

The conclusion must be, quite simply, that people benefit from what they believe in and trust. There is, in fact, no absolute distinction between a true effect—that is, the operation of a medicine—and a placebo effect; or rather, a placebo effect is a component of every true effect. It is an objective fact, proved by many tests, that aspirin is an effective treatment for headaches, but it is also a fact that many people feel the headaches easing as soon as they swallow the tablet, before the aspirin can be absorbed in the bloodstream and start working.

Just as real as the placebo effect is the nocebo effect—from the Latin *nocebo*, "I will harm." If a therapist administering a medicine warns that it may produce nausea, the expectation on the patient's part often makes it more likely that this will happen. Whether the possible side effect should be mentioned or not is a difficult problem for a doctor, but the answer depends on the degree to which the patient is accepted as "a member of the team."

What we need in this context is a thorough understanding of the concept of probability. If you press a light switch, there is a high probability that the light will come on and a low probability that it will fail to do so because the bulb is worn out, or you have forgotten to pay the electricity bill, or there is a citywide breakdown. The probability that you will suffer pain in certain circumstances, and find relief from pain in other circumstances, can also be expressed in mathematical terms, but is infinitely more difficult to predict because of the many factors involved and the variation from one individual to another. A general anesthetic is virtually certain to achieve its purpose because the power of the chemicals injected into the bloodstream far exceeds the brain's capacity to counteract them. But a procedure designed to produce analgesia—that is, absence of pain while consciousness and other functions are unaffected—is less certain to succeed, because the forces generating and neutralizing pain are more evenly balanced. As we consider various treatments, we shall see that none of them can be rated with a 100% guarantee of effectiveness. Of course, it does not follow that we should dismiss any of them as useless, or resign ourselves to the inevitability of pain. It does follow, however, that in an individual case, we may need to try various types of treatment pragmatically, and especially to combine them.

In the eighteenth century—the self-styled "age of reason"—the French Academy appointed a commission (one member was Benjamin Franklin, the American envoy in Paris) to report on mesmerism, or hypnosis as we now call it. The commission recommended the rejection of mesmerism because it had no logical rationale. But to reject a therapy because we don't understand how it achieves its effect is to put the cart before the horse. It can also, by excluding the therapy from the repertoire of qualified physicians, transfer it to the hands of unqualified practitioners, cranks, or even confidence tricksters. In our own times—bearing in mind the widespread disillusionment with orthodox medicine, particularly with regard to pain—this is a risk of which we should be keenly aware.

To search for a single treatment that could magically switch off the pain circuit would be to pursue an impossible objective. We can say this for several reasons, one being that (as we have shown earlier) there is no pain circuit, in the sense of an alarm system that could be ripped out of the body structure as a fire-alarm system might be ripped out of a building. Also, there can be no single treatment for pain, because pain itself is not a single phenomenon; it is related to various conditions of injury, tenderness, inability to move, and so forth. If we can alleviate any of these conditions, we have achieved something worthwhile. When a bedridden patient is enabled to walk, even if he experiences no change in the intensity of pain, a victory has been won.

SIDE EFFECTS

We shall soon enter in some detail into the subject of medicinal drugs, which are the best treatment for pain in millions of cases. It would be illogical to expect that the entry into the human body of a powerful chemical compound (whether of natural origin or synthetic) could have only one effect. The compound is much more likely to have side effects, which are of no value and which may in themselves be unpleasant and undesirable. This is not a reason to reject drugs in principle, but it is a reason to be aware that benefit and cost always need to be balanced. Fortunately, the side effects of the drugs we are to discuss appear gradually and are reversible, so the equation can be considered calmly. It is also true that all surgery has side effects (and these may sometimes be irreversible if some part of the body has been removed). In the Memorial Sloan–Kettering Cancer Center, the leading cancer hospital in New York, an analysis showed that 20% of the cases of patients suffering pain could be attributed to effects of treatment. There had (one hopes) been a carefully balanced consideration of the chances of prolonging life at the expense of causing pain. Both patient and therapist have an obligation to examine possible benefits and risks. Naturally, this is easier said than done, especially when a desperate patient is driven by his misery into feeling that any risk is worth taking. Hence the desirability of a second opinion—or third or fourth opinions—from medical advisers and also from the family and friends, which can assist in arriving at a rationally balanced decision.

The need for a balance between benefit and cost, or sometimes between benefit and risk, is the strongest argument for informed discussion between doctor and patient. But when both doctor and patient lock themselves into an obsessional certainty of what is the right treatment, they are giving up the open-minded quest for effective therapy or combinations of therapy. Sadly, fanatical dedication to a cult is not the monopoly of the uneducated.

A NOTE ON NAMES

Patients and doctors may well be confused by the numerous polysyllabic names of drugs. Every drug has two names—the generic or scientific name given to it when first discovered, and the brand name used for marketing purposes. The point may be illustrated by a brief history of the most common of all analgesics, or pain-killing drugs.

In 1763, the Rev. Edmund Stone of Chipping Norton wrote to the Royal Society: "There is a bark of an English tree which I have found very efficacious in curing agues and intermitting disorders." The tree in question was the willow, whose Latin name is *salix*. Chemicals derived from this tree are known scientifically as the salicylates. In 1898, a German chemist named Heinrich Dreser, working for the Bayer Company, synthesized a salicylate in a form suitable for large-scale manufacture. Its scientific name is acetylsalicylic acid but the company gave it the name of "aspirin." Today, in the United States alone, 9000 tons of aspirin are consumed in a year, or 45 million tablets every day.

There are now 12 generic names for medicines containing a salicylate or an allied substance. Collectively, they are known as nonsteroidal anti-inflammatory drugs (NSAIDs), and we shall shortly describe their properties and effects. The generic names are:

1. *Very common drugs*: acetaminophen, acetylsalicylic acid.

2. *Proprionic acids*: ibuprofen, napronen, fenoprofen, fenbufen, ketoprofen.
3. *Others*: indomethacin, ketorolac, diclofenac, mefanamic acid, pironicam.

It's worthwhile for the layman to know these names, which must by law appear on the label of the bottle (although usually in very small print). However, they are actually sold under other names, which simply indicate that they are the product of a particular company. The scientific difference between company A's ibuprofen and company B's ibuprofen is nil. The British doctor's prescription list contains 33 names for NSAIDs, and others are available over the counter without prescription. The American or French doctor's prescription list contains different company names, but the scientific names are the same. Travelers should therefore carry scientific names of their medicines. The origin of this chaos of multiple names is the commercial interest of pharmaceutical companies. They wish to link drug names and company names and to maximize their share of the market. This is done by advertising campaigns, which add to the cost of drugs. In counteraction, smaller, anonymous companies sell well-established drugs at a much cheaper rate under their scientific names. The large companies object on the grounds that the small companies have not paid for the research that invented the compound in the first place. While this socioeconomic battle continues, we take the same drug with different names and different prices.

NONNARCOTIC ANALGESICS

Nonsteroidal Anti-Inflammatory Drugs

These drugs are, by a wide margin, the most commonly used of all analgesic medicines. Their primary action is in the periphery, where they interrupt a vital stage in the inflammatory process—the production of prostaglandins, which trigger the characteristic aspects of inflammation, including heat, redness, swelling, and pain. The analgesic action is entirely in the body tissues, not in the brain. However, these drugs probably reduce fever by an impact on the hypothalamus, the part of the brain that regulates body temperature. Millions of people suffering from headaches, from arthritis, or from neuromuscular pains use these drugs, either regularly or in case of need.

Most NSAIDs are so safe that they can be bought without a prescription. Some are, in fact, mixed cocktails; the chemical composition has been altered to increase the effectiveness or to reduce undesirable side effects. For example, Bufferin is the trade name of aspirin mixed with an antacid. A very common mixture is a compound of acetaminophen or acetylsalicylic acid, with a dash of caffeine. Another trade name for a variant on aspirin is Alka-Seltzer, the long-established remedy for hangovers. NSAIDs are not narcotics, but because their effectiveness is limited and they are unequal to cope with severe pain, relatively weak narcotics—such as codeine, hydrocodeine, oxycodone, or propoxyphene—are often added to them. This generates another collection of brand names, such as Veganin and Excedrin. The narcotic element in such a drug is mild enough to permit its sale over the counter.

The drugs are being continually refined and modified by pharmaceutical research. The object of this research (in addition, of course, to putting new varieties on the market and maximizing company profits) is to increase the effectiveness of a basically weak analgesic without increasing the dangers. Take, for example, the problem of blood clots. In normal health, blood is always on the verge of clotting but is prevented from doing so by counteracting processes. When tissue damage occurs, the blood spilled into the tissue will form clots. This process is counteracted by salicylate drugs; thus, taking aspirin after a heart attack or a stroke reduces the danger of blood vessels forming further clots. That's the good news. The bad news is that some parts of the body, such as the gastrointestinal tract, have a tendency to bleed all the time (even in the absence of an ulcer or similar ailment) and therefore require a certain amount of clotting. Thus, ingestion of aspirin may lead to the appearance of small amounts of blood in the feces. In sensitive people, the reaction takes the form of nausea, vomiting, and dyspepsia (commonly called indigestion).

An individual with a finely tuned immune system may develop violent allergic reactions to drugs that the body recognizes as foreign invaders. These reactions seldom occur in the average person. But because these drugs are easily available and are not thought of as threatening, people tend to think that four aspirins will do twice as much good as two aspirins, and they consume dangerously toxic quantities. Also, some people fail to appreciate the dangers of consuming inappropriate mixtures of chemical compounds. The comic stage drunk has a red nose and a hiccup: the red nose because alcohol dilates the blood vessels and a hiccup because it irritates the stomach lining. The real drunk totters to the bathroom and adds aspirin to his stomach contents in the hope of stopping the oncoming hangover. The alcohol and the aspirin cooperate in their attack on the stomach, which produces the most common cause of violent gastric hemorrhage.

The truth is—and we can do nothing about it—that any increase in the effectiveness of a drug leads to an increase in the seriousness of the side effects. Acetominophen, a very mild drug, has almost no side effects at normal dosage, but it also has very little anti-inflammatory action. A highly effective drug can have absolutely unacceptable side effects, and this is why some NSAIDs—zomepirac, benoxoprofen, suprofen—have been banned by governmental action. All that the individual pain sufferer can do, in consultation with the doctor, is to make a rational balance between the good and the bad and seek, by trial and error, the drug that best suits his constitution.

STEROIDS

Steroid drugs (as distinct from nonsteroids) are extremely powerful compounds, related to naturally produced hormones, which control reaction to injury at a more fundamental level than the NSAIDs. Cortisone is an example of a steroid drug. The therapeutic effects are dramatic; so are the dangers. Therefore, steroids are used with great caution. If a steroid is applied to the body as a whole, the most usual practice is to apply it briefly to bring a near-lethal condition under control.

A good example of the delicate balance required in therapy concerns inflammation. Of course, it is a harmful process which we wish to combat, but the body needs the capacity to make small inflammatory responses in order to repel bacterial invasions. The loss of this capacity could be equivalent to destruction of the immune system, as in AIDS, and would invite infection by all sorts of bacterial organisms. If we use a steroid against inflammation and wipe out this beneficial aspect of inflammation, we could obviously do more harm than good.

The big advantage of steroid drugs is that their great power enables us to target them on the exact point of the desired action, while avoiding any application to the body as a whole. If this is done, the harmful effects are not generalized. It is possible to soak a section of skin, or even the conjunctiva of the eye, in steroids. A deeper structure, such as a joint, can be injected with a concentrated small volume of the drug, which will leak slowly onto nearby tissue. Researchers in this field are constantly seeking to find more and more subtle ways of using this localized targeting process.

LOCAL ANESTHETICS

Imagine a chemical so powerful that it could not be used in general anesthesia without killing the patient, but is ideally suited to targeted therapy and local anesthesia. A century ago, it was discovered that such a chemical could be derived from an herb occurring in nature—coca. Two Viennese physicians, Sigmund Freud and Carl Koller, made the first investigation of the effects of cocaine, in 1884. Freud was fascinated by its action on the central nervous system and its application to all kinds of disorders of the mind and body; he used it to wean a colleague from morphine addiction, but unfortunately turned the man into a cocaine addict. Koller concentrated on the peripheral action of cocaine and succeeded in anesthetizing the eye with cocaine drops. The significance of this feat was quickly recognized. Within a year, by 1885, Hall had already used cocaine for dental anesthesia.

At this time, The Johns Hopkins Hospital in Baltimore had just opened, with a galaxy of talent, leading the world in medical and surgical innovation. It is therefore no surprise that Halsted, the Professor of Surgery, introduced local nerve blocks for anesthesia in surgery in 1885. In their enthusiasm to investigate how to block different nerves, Halsted and his colleagues experimented on themselves. In the process, several of them became lifelong cocaine addicts, which did not prevent them from becoming the most influential professors of surgery in their day. By 1885, Corning had applied cocaine directly to the spinal cord. A tragicomic aspect of the first case of spinal anesthesia was that the patient was being treated for masturbation, then regarded as a grave medical problem. Cocaine treatment for this problem did not flourish, but the technique has been universally developed for more serious purposes.

Exploration of anesthetic techniques is still being pursued today, mainly in two directions. One is development of skills by anesthesiologists to insert needles and catheters so that they can flood particular nerves or nerve roots. The other is modification of the cocaine molecule to prolong its effect, increase its stability, and reduce undesirable effects—in particular, its psychedelic action. This has generated a family of compounds with names ending in -caine, including procaine, novocaine, lidocaine, and bupivecaine.

How does a local anesthetic work? Excitable tissue, whether muscle or a nerve, can generate a wave of sudden change. In the case of a nerve, this change takes the form of an impulse that travels from one end of a nerve cell to the other and carries the message that the cell has been stimulated. The disturbance consists of the very rapid opening of channels which allow ions such as sodium or potassium to rush from one side of the membrane. Cocaine prevents one of these channels from opening and thereby blocks the impulse. The membrane is stabilized and cannot break down to generate nerve impulses.

As we might expect, there are some undesirable side effects. A nerve contains a mixture of sensory and motor nerve fibers. If we bring about a complete blockage of all sensory input—that is, anesthesia and not merely analgesia—we inevitably block the motor fibers too and thus cause paralysis, as experienced by anyone having a dental local anesthetic. Let us recall the use of local anesthesia as a spinal block during childbirth. The mother is anesthetized in parts of her body that might be painful, while the baby is unaffected (and the mother remains conscious) because the bloodstream is absorbing only a minute quantity of the drug. The cost accompanying this benefit is that the motor fibers are blocked when the dose is high so that the legs are weak. Furthermore, the anesthetized part of the spinal cord contains output nerve fibers leading to the viscera and to the blood vessels in the legs and abdomen. The result is temporary incontinence and loss of the ability to constrict blood vessels and maintain blood pressure if the mother stands. Fortunately, these side effects are transient and reversible and are worth tolerating in view of the advantages.

Local anesthesia can be maintained for hours, or even days, by giving small top-up doses. This is often done to alleviate postoperative pain or after severe accidents involving the legs and the pelvis. But it is unwise to continue the anesthesia indefinitely because new side effects appear. The drugs block the supply of chemicals from the nerve cell body which provides distant parts of the nerves with vital nourishment. Interrupting this process for a limited time does no harm, but the nerve fibers could ultimately decay from starvation. Should this happen, the effect would be the same as though the nerve had been cut. Current research has the aim of preventing this dangerous side effect, or possibly turning it to advantage.

ANTISYMPATHETIC THERAPY

The sympathetic system, a specialized part of the nervous system that regulates the activity of tissues, originates in a chain of ganglia positioned on either side of the spinal column (see Fig. 6). Nerve fibers from these ganglia emit chemicals, such as norepinephrine, which control, among other things, the diameter of blood vessels. Normally, the action of these fibers has no effect on sensation, but when nerves are damaged they become sensitive to sympathetic action, causing some of the most terrible pains that human beings can experience. It is possible to relieve this pain by stopping the action of sympathetic nerves. The problem is that since every part of the body depends on continuous regulation, putting the whole sympathetic system into suspension would be a blunderbuss remedy causing all kinds of harmful consequences. For instance, impotence and incontinence follow if control of the pelvic viscera is lost. If blood vessels in the legs cease to constrict in the normal way, the person thus affected cannot stand without fainting. Clearly, therapy directed at the sympathetic nerves requires targeting.

There are several ways of doing this. The ganglia that cause pain can be destroyed, either by open surgery or by local injection with a chemical to destroy the nerve cells. Another method, suitable when the pain is in an arm or leg, is to close off the blood vessels to the limb with a blood pressure cuff, which is a safe procedure for a limited time, and inject a chemical that temporarily destroys the endings of the sympathetic nerves. When the cuff is removed and circulation resumes, the chemical is so diluted that it has no effect on the rest of the body. A third method, extremely subtle and just recently being explored, is to inject highly selective blocking agents that affect only the sensitizing action of the sympathetic nerves and leave other functions intact. Altogether, antisympathetic therapy is a fine example of a specialized remedy for a particular type of pain and has proved highly successful.

ANTIDEPRESSANTS

Although individuals vary greatly in courage and morale, chronic pain is inevitably a depressing experience. Worse, it contributes to a downward spiral; pain increases depression, which increases pain. Counteracting depression, therefore, is an integral part of the treatment of pain. Our most obvious resources are antidepressant drugs, available in two families: tricyclic drugs, of which amitryptyline and imipramine are the best known, and monoamine oxidase inhibitors, of which phenelzine is the most common.

When these drugs were first used, a lucky and exciting discovery was made. In addition to their antidepressant function, they directly relieve pain. They do this by raising the concentration in the brain of a group of neurotransmitters, such as dopamine, noradrenaline, and serotonin, which generate some of the inhibitory components of gate control. It has been observed that the analgesic or pain-relieving action occurs within 3 to 7 days, whereas the relief of depression requires 2 or 3 weeks. Also, the analgesic action is in evidence when antidepressant drugs are given to patients who are not depressed. The drugs have been used successfully in a variety of painful conditions, including arthritis, cancer, and neuropathies. Their most welcome function is to relieve the otherwise untreatable pain that occurs when sensory nerves are damaged by disease. One such condition is diabetes; another is postherpetic neuralgia following an attack of shingles. Sometimes, these drugs are used in combination with major tranquilizers for a brief period to regain control over pain. There are no dangerous side effects.

OPIATES, OR NARCOTIC ANALGESICS

In Homer's *Odyssey*, Helen dispensed a delectable substance "to lull all pain and anger and bring forgetfulness of every sorrow." It was opium, easily derived from a common variety of poppy. Opium is described, always favorably, in ancient writings in Sumeria, Egypt, and China. Galen, the Roman Empire's leading medical authority, recommended it as a cure for "deafness, epilepsy, fevers, the troubles to which women are subject, melancholy, and all pestilence."

Sir Thomas Sydenham, an English doctor, wrote in 1680: "Among the remedies which it has pleased Almighty God to give to man to relieve his sufferings, none is so universal and so efficacious as opium." By this time, people who had taken opium to relieve pain found that it was a source of positive pleasure and kept up the habit as an indulgence in good health. Medical texts began to contain warnings that excessive use of opium could be harmful or even fatal. Robert Clive, the conqueror of India, took opium steadily for 20 years and is said to have died of a fit after taking a double dose (although it may be that he committed suicide to evade charges of extortion and corruption).

Opium reached its peak of popularity in the nineteenth century; it was easily available and indulgence carried no stigma. When Marx called religion "the opium of the people," he meant that it was comforting. Thomas De Quincey's *Confessions of an English Opium Eater* was a best-seller, and frequent or occasional users included Byron, Shelley, Keats, Coleridge, Dickens, Turner, Darwin—and Florence Nightingale. Under the British Raj, the growing of opium in India was encouraged and two aggressive wars were launched to compel China, the first nation to regard opium as a threat, to import the surplus production. Among officials employed in the Raj's Opium Department—which existed to make opium-growing more efficient, not to suppress it—was George Orwell's father, who retired in 1912.

Meanwhile, chemists were at work to synthesize opium derivatives that had greater strength with less bulk and could be given to patients by injection. Morphine—named after Morpheus, the god of sleep, because it relieved insomnia—was produced as early as 1803. In 1874, this was followed by the stronger diamorphine. This drug was first marketed commercially by the Bayer Company, which we have already cited as the pioneer of aspirin. The company's sales department (or promotion department) triumphantly claimed that it was as strong as a legendary hero and named it heroin. In fact, while morphine is 10 times as strong as natural opium resin, heroin is 25 times as strong.

Opium contains two other analgesics, codeine and thebaine, and also an unrelated chemical, papaverine, which relaxes smooth muscle and dilates blood vessels. We now have a large number of drugs of this type. They are known as narcotics, from a Greek word meaning "to numb or stupefy." They vary considerably in their potency, the duration of the effect, and the possible side effects, and the suitability of a drug for an individual patient has to be decided according to his characteristics. We give a very short list of the most commonly used narcotics:

Generic name	Some trade names
Weak narcotics	
Codeine	(sold as codeine)
Dihydrocodeine	Paracodin (U.S.); DF 118 (U.K.)
Oxycodone	Percodan
Dextropropoxyphine	Darvon (U.S.); Distalgesic (U.K.)
Strong narcotics	
Morphine	(prescribed as morphine)
Diacetylmorphine	Heroin
Methadone	Dalophine (U.S.); Physeptone (U.K.)
Pethidine	Demerol (U.S.)
Buprenorphine	Temgesic
Hydromorphone	Dilaudid
Levorphonol	Dromoran

Helen of Troy, Galen, and Sir Thomas Sydenham were not wrong; narcotic drugs are extremely efficient in the relief of pain, as millions of sufferers and many thousands of doctors could testify. The World Health Organization has initiated a campaign to make these drugs more widely available and to combat the confusion and ignorance that limit their use. On the other hand, some governments, notably the United States, are vigorously seeking to prevent access to strong narcotics such as heroin. Once the sale of heroin was made illegal, the trade predictably fell into the hands of highly organized, resourceful criminal gangs, like the trade in alcohol during Prohibition. Regrettable though it may appear, opium growers and traders in such countries as Burma or Pakistan do not feel that they are engaged in a more evil activity than distillers who produce whisky in Scotland.

This subject is difficult to discuss unemotionally. Since the 1960s, addiction to heroin, and in more recent years to cocaine or "crack," has reached epidemic proportions in some parts of major American cities. The limitless indulgence to which the addict is prone is extremely harmful to the human organism and can lead to an early death; many are the tragedies for which it can be justly blamed. Moreover, there is an obvious link between the world of addiction and the world of crime, and drugs are a factor in causing a large proportion of murders, muggings, and thefts, which have inexorably become more numerous year by year. Clearly, we are faced with a very grave social problem, and the authors of this book are in no way inclined to dismiss or minimize it.

However, it is necessary to draw a firm distinction between the beneficial use of narcotics—primarily to combat pain—and their excessive, unregulated use for psychedelic or conscious-ness-changing purposes. The sufferer from pain who accepts a narcotic is motivated, quite simply and reasonably, by a desire to relieve the pain. Rather than grouping the heroin addict with such a person, it is more logical to group him with addicts to alcohol, tobacco, betel-nut chewing, or any other habit that can become compulsive. Heroin itself is neither good nor bad; what makes it good—or bad—is the purpose and context of the usage.

Hence, certain widely accepted beliefs call for reexamination. First, it is believed that narcotics given in doses strong enough to stop pain will kill the patient by respiratory depression. This is simply untrue; on the contrary, the correct use of morphine, by freeing the patient from pain, renders him more capable of sleeping, eating, and moving in a natural way, and thus prolongs his life.

Second, it is believed that tolerance of the drug—that is, a process whereby a stated dose becomes ineffective and stronger doses are demanded—necessarily develops so rapidly that control cannot be maintained. In reality, no such problem arises when opiates are given steadily to relieve chronic pain. Indeed, the patient whose pain has been successfully relieved often voluntarily asks to be given weaker or less frequent doses. It is the addict who changes his tolerance and requires stronger doses to get his kick, and the reason lies in his addiction, not in the nature of narcotic drugs. Similarly, alcoholics demand ever-greater quantities of liquor as their addiction grows more severe, while ordinary people go on year after year consuming the same selected amount of wine or beer.

Third, there is the belief that any intake of narcotics leads inevitably to helpless addiction. It is because of this belief that the use of heroin in hospitals is outlawed in some American states. There have, it is true, been cases of hospital patients who received heroin and went on to seek it in the outside world (and also cases of doctors who developed the heroin habit through their authorized access), but these are few and far between among the, unfortunately, far greater numbers of people who were introduced to heroin "on the street." What needs to be emphasized is that the overwhelming majority of patients receiving heroin see it as part of the hospital experience and are finished with it when they are finished with that experience. This fact refutes the theory of inevitable addiction, and also justifies—if justification is needed—the medicinal use of narcotics.

Indeed, even a person who indulges in narcotic drugs as a pleasure, or out of curiosity, does not necessarily become an addict. We have noted that in the nineteenth century, before illegalization drove drug users into a social ghetto, people were taking opium as they desired it and keeping it under control. Today, it is estimated that about four million Americans take heroin at one time or another—perhaps for pleasure, perhaps to relieve chronic pain—of whom half a million are addicts. And while we are rightly concerned about the scourge of addiction, we tend to forget the more comforting fact that thousands of young people have experimented with drugs and—whether through growing maturity, the need to hold down a job, or moving into a different social circle—have brought the experiment to a halt.

We now return to the subject of the use of opiates to relieve pain. They are not a panacea for every kind of pain; clearly, there is no such panacea. They do not work on certain types of chronic pain involving nerve damage. They work best, and indeed are immensely effective, in cases of postoperative pain and of pain related to cancer. To understand why they are useful in some contexts but not others, we have to understand how they operate. They act on the central nervous system (this has been proved by the application of very small amounts directly on the brain) because structures in this system generate proteins that are receptors specific to narcotics. The reason for the existence of these receptors is that the brain produces its own opiates, which then interact with the receptors.

These endogenous opiates belong to three classes: endorphins, dynorphins, and enkephalins. Rather like a pharmaceutical company, the brain produces a variety of opiates serving different purposes (although, unlike a pharmaceutical company, it doesn't produce an identical opiate with a new name). All reactions caused by endogenous opiates are natural and desirable when occurring at relevant times and relevant places.

But reactions caused by external opiates—that is, drugs—include desirable and undesirable effects. The desirable effect, of course, is analgesia. In order to secure this effect and avoid others, we must seek to target the drug.

One way in which this is being attempted, so far with little success, is to search for opiates that interact only with subsets of the receptors. This field of research is partly responsible for the very large number of available narcotics. Heroin, in fact, was originally synthesized in an attempt to separate analgesia from addiction.

Another approach has been much more successful. This was a search for the zone within the brain where the analgesia-producing action is generated. Through injections of minute amounts of morphine, such a zone was detected in the mid-brain. When electrically stimulated, it produced analgesia by means of descending impulses directed at the gate control in the spinal cord. Unfortunately, to place morphine in this region and this region alone is not practicable, although stimulating electrodes have been installed in a number of patients. However, a second zone sensitive to narcotics was discovered in the dorsal horn—at the spot where the gate control operates. To apply drugs directly to the spinal cord is quite easy. It was found that morphine applied locally produced analgesia limited to the segments treated. It was not even necessary to puncture the dura with a needle, for the same effect could be achieved outside the meninges with an epidural catheter of the type used for local anesthetics. This has now become common practice. The discovery of the sensitive zone also led to an understanding of why narcotic drugs are ineffective against nerve deafferentation pains. Opiate receptors disappear in deafferentation, so an essential condition for the action of a narcotic is absent.

Progress is also being made in studying and controlling the time course of narcotic action. Preventing the onset of pain requires a much smaller dose than combating it after it is established. Thus, drugs to stop postoperative pain can be safely given before the operation instead of afterward. Patients need no longer alternate between analgesia and spells of intolerable pain.

Narcotics work best when given in frequent doses or continuously, but frequent injections are desired neither by the patient who wants to rest and sleep nor by the busy hospital staff. Simple gadgetry has been developed to allow either intermittent injection or continuous steady injection. With growing confidence that these methods are effective and safe, the idea of allowing the patient to control his own analgesia grew up. It is called patient-controlled analgesia, or PCA. Drugs formerly regarded as dangerous or addictive, and hence inadequately given, are now entrusted to the patient's own judgment. It has been most interesting to see what happens. The mechanical gadgets have safeguards to check overuse, but in practice no patient even approaches the limits. On the contrary, most patients allow themselves a smaller overall dose than the staff would have administered under the old system. They reduce the pain to a bearable level, but refrain from drugging themselves to a degree that would prevent them from thinking clearly. Control and choice—the essentials of being human—are never lost. The patient is never plunged into utter helplessness and total dependence on others. This in itself is an important contribution to limiting the misery of serious illness, and even the ultimate fear of death.

But the value of narcotic drugs should not allow us to leave the existence of side effects out of account. When the drugs are first administered, they leave the patient drowsy and mentally confused. Fortunately, the brain develops a tolerance, which causes this effect to disappear while analgesia is maintained. This is not the same as the kind of tolerance that drives the addict to venture on higher and higher intakes. The patient can adjust to a steady, consistent level of drug use while recovering from the side effect.

Another common side effect has a curious origin. The body's endogenous opiates do not occur only in the nervous system. Some nerve cells in the gut release opiates that affect nearby receptors. When narcotic drugs are given, they affect this mechanism, resulting in nausea, vomiting, and constipation. These side effects, although unpleasant, can be brought under control by simple, well-known remedies.

The battle for constructive use of narcotics was not easy to wage, nor is it entirely won. It involves hard questioning, intensive investigation, and confrontation with obstinate dogmas. Progress in scientific knowledge and good medical practice is one thing; the reeducation of doctors, patients, and an entire social environment is something else.

ANTIEPILEPTIC DRUGS

Before leaving this field, we should mention a type of drug appropriate to a particular and unusual type of pain. Groups of sensory nerve cells in the dorsal horn (or in its equivalent in the medulla) can reach a level of extreme excitability so that they fire impulses in an explosive burst. Sad to say, this occurs particularly in the nerves that serve the face. The firing can occur in response to a light and normally innocuous stimulus of the skin, or even spontaneously. The most common of these conditions is trigeminal neuralgia, in which the sufferer experiences sudden jolting stabs of pain in the face for no apparent reason. This condition has something in common with epilepsy, which is caused by the firing of nerve cells in the cerebral cortex. Drugs used in treating epilepsy (one of these is carbamazepine, with the trade name of Tegretol) work by decreasing the excitability of nerve cells, so it seems logical that the same drugs should have a sedative and pain-relieving effect on patients with trigeminal neuralgia, and they generally do. Sometimes, however, the stabs of pain cannot be brought fully under control or the sedation is unacceptable, and in these cases the one remaining resource is surgery.

We have described seven classes of medicine used against pain:

1. Aspirin and compounds with aspirin
2. Steroids
3. Antidepressants
4. Antisympathetic drugs
5. Local anesthetics
6. Narcotics
7. Antiepileptics

Each of these succeeds in controlling a particular type of pain. Each has side effects, which must be balanced against the undoubted benefits. One method of improving effectiveness is to target the medicine onto the precise point of its beneficial action. Another method is to involve the patient in his own treatment. The development of these drugs has been an enormous boon for people afflicted by pain. But our description of the resources that can now be mobilized in the fight against pain is not yet complete; it will require two more chapters.

9

Therapy by Surgery, Restoration, or Stimulation

Many patients may have an overwhelming conviction that their pain is caused by something inside them which should be cut out by a surgeon. They may be right. Operations to remove kidney stones or cancer blocking the bowel or arthritic hip joints can be spectacularly successful. The high profile of such surgery encourages a belief that all pains should be curable by surgery. This is unfortunately wrong. It is true that surgeons have the means to numb any part of the body by making nerve lesions, but while this is fully justified on occasions, it does not dispose of all long-term problems. There is also the common-sense belief that some pains must be caused by mechanical pressures and tensions. This is also true on occasions that we will describe. These conditions may be successfully treated by orthopedic surgery and less intrusively by osteopaths and chiropractors.

The third group of therapies to be described in this chapter may be more surprising in their rationale. They all involve doing something active to the patient, which results in generating more nerve impulses. The explanation for their success depends on the recognition that pain mechanisms are dynamic, with the body containing its own mechanisms, such as the gate control, which can increase and decrease pain. Some of these treatments are centuries old, but they gain more respect as the reasons for their success become apparent and hence achieve further development. Because this book is concerned with people with ongoing pains, we do not discuss those special and fortunate cases in which an immediate and complete cure is feasible.

SURGERY

Surgery that Cuts Nerves, Roots, or Tracts

There are two ways to cut peripheral nerves or central nerve tracts. One is the classical method of open surgery, in which the structure is exposed and cut. Because this involves major surgery with all its advantages and dangers, a great deal of ingenuity has been used to push long needles through the skin until the tip rests against the nerve or tract that is to be destroyed. The general location of the tip and target structure are known because we are all approximately the same anatomically. This is particularly impressive in the brain, for which three-dimensional maps have been made that allow the stereotactic position of each brain area to be located with respect to landmarks on the skull. Once the tip is in the correct general position, its precise position is adjusted by X-ray techniques, by making recordings of nerve impulses, or by using the tip itself as a stimulating electrode. Then the lesion can be made, either by electrically heating the tip or by injecting chemicals.

The basic rationale for such an operation derived from the classical idea of pain fibers, pain pathways, and a pain center. As we explained before, we now understand pain as a phenomenon depending on a balance of excitatory and inhibitory actions. This new understanding explains why surgery often led to only temporary relief and was sometimes followed by other painful feelings produced by the deafferentation, which can itself produce problems. So, despite all the skill and high technology developed to make this type of surgery feasible, its use is decreasing and is limited to certain special circumstances. However, even when we know that the surgery will bring only temporary benefit and will eventually cause other undesirable symptoms, it can be fully justified in bringing relief from pain to a patient who has not long to live.

The Trigeminal Nerve. Trigeminal neuralgia, the violent stabs of face pain we described earlier, can be eliminated if the trigeminal nerve is cut. The sensory nerve fibers that trigger the pain converge onto a ganglion that lies in the base of the skull just in front of the ear. This can be exposed by open surgery or reached by needles pushed through the foramina in the skull, the holes through which the nerves run to reach the face. Destruction of the whole nerve leaves the patient with the feeling of a numb face and also deprives the eye of its protective blinking reflex. The surgeon tries, therefore, to cut only those nerve fibers which come from the trigger zone. Trigeminal neuralgia, although horribly painful, is strictly localized. Thus, a small reduction of the nerve impulses, either by cutting the fiber or by injecting a chemical such as glycerol, can make all the difference. The operation is delicate but not complicated. It is used for those patients who don't respond to caramazepine. The disease may return, but in that case the operation can be repeated.

Roots. Destroying an entire nerve root is a drastic procedure, not often carried out nowadays because of the high rate of recurrence of pain and the very unpleasant consequences of deafferentation. However, selective partial lesions are still in the neurosurgeon's repertoire. Such an operation is particularly suitable for a patient with pain in the leg or pelvis and a short life expectancy. The most common method is to place a pool of the nerve fiber–destroying chemical, phenol, around the roots to be destroyed.

Dorsal Horn. Brachial plexus avulsion is a tragic condition that has become common in victims of motorcycle accidents. If thrown from his machine, the rider has his head protected by his helmet, but his shoulder is violently dislocated when it hits the ground. The nerve roots entering the spinal cord may be wrenched out, leaving the patient with a completely paralyzed arm. Because all the afferent nerves have been destroyed, and the cells of the dorsal horn are freed for unlimited excitability, the result is an extreme level of burning, continuous deafferentation pain. Drugs give no relief, so a relatively new operation on the dorsal root entry zone has been developed. The affected part of the spinal cord is exposed and needles are placed in the entire length of the dorsal horn to kill the deafferented cells by a series of heat lesions.

There is not yet enough evidence for a verdict on this procedure, but one case is worth describing. The patient had a paralyzed arm, completely devoid of feeling, before the operation and this condition persisted afterward. But the hyperexcitable cells which had been attempting to overcome the loss of sensory input, thus generating the continuous pain, were destroyed, and so the pain was eliminated.

Cordotomy. In the nineteenth century it was observed that if the ventral quadrant of the spinal cord had been destroyed by injury or disease, the patient could not feel a pinprick or a change in temperature on the opposite side of the body below the lesion. This led to the idea of making the lesion deliberately to relieve pain in the lower torso or the leg. The operation can be carried out either by open surgery or by inserting a needle through the gap between the vertebrae in the neck. Pain is indeed relieved, but the effect fades after some months and repeat operations are unsuccessful. Therefore, this operation is now considered appropriate only for patients who have a short time to live. Another disadvantage is that if the pain is felt on both sides of the body and the operation therefore must be done on both sides, the aftereffects may include motor weakness, urinary dysfunction, and dysesthesia (an unpleasant feeling in all sensation). All these operations have become less common as the knowledge of how to use analgesic medicine has improved.

Psychosurgery

We now come to a type of surgery based on a distinctive rationale: the idea that it should be possible to sever the parts of the brain responsible for the interpretation of pain sensations. The relevant parts were thought to be in the frontal and limbic areas. In 1973, a famous pain surgeon expressed the view that this surgery was justified when a patient exhibited "an excessive and futile emotional response to pain." This attitude implies a distinction between pain itself and the response, or between sensation and perception—distinctions that, as we have stressed throughout this book, do not exist. It also assumes the right of some judgmental authority, presumably a senior medical figure, to condemn the patient's behavior as excessive and futile.

Nineteen different types of psychosurgery have been used, starting with the original complete bilateral frontal lobotomy of 1936 and moving to much more limited, discrete operations which produce much less personality demolition. Attempts to produce the desired effect by lesions in various parts of the thalamus were tried, but abandoned because of the high rate of recurrence, speech difficulties, unpleasant sensations, and even mortality. For the large frontal lobotomies, despite success in the relief of suffering for a short period, psychological deterioration was a major problem. Dr. A. J. Bouckoms of the Massachusetts General Hospital in Boston has summarized the present status of psychosurgery for pain in his chapter in the *Textbook of Pain* listed in the Further Reading section at the end of this volume. He describes the deterioration following the large frontal lobotomies as commonly including excessive masturbation, disorientation, incontinence, and unruly behavior.

From the 1960s these large lesions were replaced by smaller cuts restricted to the most medial posterior part of the frontal lobe. He concludes that these lesions produce a clear short-term benefit in 50–75% of the patients but the longer-term benefits are more equivocal because there is mental deterioration in 10–30% of the patients. The surgeon who is confronted by an anxious, terrified patient in pain is tempted to use desperate measures in such a desperate situation. Such decisions are clearly extremely difficult and both surgeon and patient need help in reaching a considered conclusion.

Surgery to Relieve Pressure

Peripheral Nerves. When nerves are trapped in scar tissue, the response on a surgeon's part is to cut them free. This intervention sometimes relieves pain; the trouble is that, if it fails, a second attempt almost always makes things worse.

Dr. C. E. Wynn-Parry, a wise British physician with great experience dealing with nerve injuries, takes the view that surgeons should be allowed one try and no more. The reason for the low success rate is that the pain-producing pathology has migrated centrally from the original site. We have described the cascade of changes that sweep into the spinal cord and beyond. If this is the case, peripheral surgery merely adds to the original damage.

The one fortunate exception is the carpal tunnel syndrome. Nerves and tendons running from the arm to the hand pass through the carpal tunnel, which is closed over by a thick band of fibrous tissue at the wrist with the function of keeping the tendons close to the wrist bones. As people grow older, the band thickens and presses on the nerves, causing pins-and-needles sensations and eventually serious pain. Cutting the band, if it is done early enough, brings immediate and complete relief.

Disc Surgery. Surgery on spinal discs was first carried out in 1933. It has come to dominate much thinking about pain in general and back pain in particular. Pressure on a nerve root seems the logical explanation for a pain and disc removal the logical answer. The ability to observe pressure on roots by discs or by bone has been greatly improved by the development of imaging techniques beyond normal X-rays. The computed axial tomography (CAT) scan allows an X-ray image to be calculated as though a slice were taken through the bone. Myelography, by filling the cerebrospinal fluid with an X-ray–dense material, makes it possible to see exactly where the roots are running. Now nuclear magnetic resonance images (NMRI) allow precise localization of different types of soft tissue in addition to bone.

It is therefore possible now to investigate the relationship between the disc and the pain. It is not obvious. Some patients with an undoubted herniated disc and with severe pain are treated conservatively with rest or traction and get better. On reexamination the disc is found to be unchanged. Many patients in pain from discs fail to show the motor signs that would be expected if roots were compressed. This suggests that the pain comes not from root compression, but from some other tissue in the region that produces a pattern of referred pain. This idea is supported by the finding that local anesthetic blocks of nerves in the leg relieve the pain, which would not happen if the "pain" impulses were being generated in the root, but would happen if the pain was of the referred variety, which we discussed in relation to the arm and chest pain of angina pectoris. The honest answer on the cause of pain in the presence of a herniated disc is that we are no more certain of the origin of the pain than we are in those 70% to 80% of low back pains where no lesion is apparent.

The popular belief that most back pain is caused by root compression by slipped discs and cured by surgery is so powerful as to be uninfluenced by the facts about cause and cure. The reported rate of surgical failure is usually 5% to 10%

but there are large variations, with some hospitals reporting more than 50% failure. In the most recent U.S. long-term follow-up of 100 patients at 5 years, 62% of the patients were pain-free, 20% were as bad as or worse than at the time of the operation, and 18% had had subsequent back surgery. There is a relationship between the short-term success and the degree of herniation, with 90% success with complete herniation to 40% success when no herniation is found. Repeat operations have a lower and lower success rate. Failure is not just a lack of success—some patients are clearly worse after surgery.

There is a very real and serious ethical, legal, and practical problem in testing the effectiveness of established therapies. A test would involve withholding an accepted treatment from a patient. Few patients in their right mind would consent to such a gamble for the sake of scientific interest. If the doctor did not operate and did not obtain the patient's willing and informed consent, he should certainly be arrested or sued or both. What has been done legally with proper consent was to take 126 patients with questionable indications for discectomy and to operate on half and give physiotherapy to the other half. After one year, the operated patients were better off, but the difference disappeared by 4 years, and after 10 years the rate of persistent low back pain in the two groups was equal.

Between hospitals, states, and countries there is a huge variation in the rate of disc removal with little evidence of a difference in the rate of long-term back pain. In certain very rare conditions (1 in 200,000 per year), emergency disc operation is surely mandatory. In less dramatic circumstances, removal of grossly herniated discs is presumably good practice, although for some it is too late to correct the damage. In less severe distortions it may be that, as with many other therapies, the intervention may bring short-term relief (provided that no accident has occurred during the surgery to make the disease worse) but makes no difference in the long run.

Orthopedic surgeons are also in the business of relieving pain by relieving pressure. As far back as 1827, a surgeon named Barton cut across a femur to correct a deformed hip. Joints and their surrounding tissue are subjected to ingenious operations to correct abnormal pressure distributions. The procedure culminates in joint replacements with artificial substitutes. After a hip replacement for painful arthritis, about one-third of the patients are pain-free and able to move well, one-third are pain-free but still very restricted in movement, and one-third are no better or indeed worse. For the vertebrae, especially with disc lesions, the orthopedic surgeon often extends the neurosurgeon's approach, which naturally concentrates on the assumed root damage; the procedure is to increase the stability of the vertebrae whose disc has collapsed and herniated by joining the vertebrae rigidly together with a bone graft. This may be compared to the work of a carpenter who restores old furniture but keeps to the spirit of the original design. The operation often works well, but is not always appropriate.

MANIPULATION TO RELIEVE PRESSURE: OSTEOPATHS AND CHIROPRACTORS

We have seen that the apparently obvious relation between slipped discs and pain is far from clear. Relief from pain may follow from disc surgery, but it may also occur without surgery or may be caused by some other effect of cutting in the region. If there is uncertainty about surgery, it is even harder to make definite statements about the rationale and effects of osteopathy and chiropractics. The theory is to ascribe the pain (and many other conditions) to misplaced vertebrae. This theory may be wrong, and certainly the enthusiasts have been unable to convince open-minded people outside their inner circle. What is important is not to debate the theory, but rather to see whether the practice works. We need controlled trials to discover just what works, when, and with which patients. The knowledge is required both to provide an understanding, and in order that patients will know what to expect. On the crassest level, it is needed to establish professional status and to persuade governments and insurance companies that they are not wasting their money.

There have been 20 controlled trials of spinal manipulation. Nine showed little or no lasting effect, while 11 did show an effect. Unlike democracy, science does not work by majority vote. During the treatment, most of the patients felt better; the problem is with the long-term results. The vituperative exchanges between rival experts on pain at international meetings would be good comedy if the subject were not so tragically real. The arguments concern the question of whether the negative and positive trials are comparable, with regard to the condition of the patients, the precise technique employed, and the end result.

To reach a conclusion will take a lot of hard work and study, involving the examination of particular techniques on particular pains. Meanwhile, there is no reason why a person in pain should not receive treatment from a qualified manipulator. It may do good and will certainly do no harm.

"MAGIC BULLETS" TO RELIEVE PRESSURE: RADIOTHERAPY AND CHEMOTHERAPY

We have described the targeted application of drugs; there are also targeted methods of reducing the size of cancers. Many cancers are selectively sensitive to X-radiation or to hormones or to anticancer drugs.

When the pains of cancer are produced by the ongoing presence of tumors that are creating pressure, it is obvious that palliative relief can be obtained by reducing the pressure. This can sometimes be done by surgery, but that is fairly rare. Some tumors shrink, although they do not disappear, if they are irradiated with X-ray beams or from radioactive sources. Similarly, some tumors are sensitive to hormones and decrease in size with hormone therapy or with destruction of the pituitary, which is the master gland of the hormone system. Tumors that are very sensitive to chemotherapy will also decrease in size after treatment with the appropriate cytotoxic compound. All these treatments have very marked side effects, and the patient and doctor must have a very open, honest discussion to match the costs with the benefits. It must also be understood that the aim is palliation, not cure.

STIMULATION THERAPY

A large number of therapies work by stimulating the nervous system, not by blocking or cutting. Once we abandon the old theory of the "pain pathway" and accept that pain is the consequence of a balance between excitatory and inhibitory processes, this makes good sense. The advantages of stimulation therapy are that it destroys nothing, it has no side effects, and it is reversible. Its effectiveness depends partly on the placebo process, but this should be welcomed.

One finding that led to the gate-control theory was the discovery that stimulation of large, low-threshold afferent nerve fibers partially inhibited the response to noxious stimuli of transmitting cells in the spinal cord. These fibers can easily be stimulated by electrical currents. One of the authors (P.D.W.), then at Massachusetts Institute of Technology, and William Sweet, Professor of Neurosurgery at Harvard, first tried the effect of gentle high-frequency electrical stimulation on their own nerves and found it effective enough to blunt the effect of a pinprick (73). They then tried the effect of inserting electrical stimulating needles close to their nerves, just as the surgeons at Johns Hopkins 70 years earlier had experimented on themselves to find out how to give local anesthesia. That was easy and interesting, but the reader can imagine the trepidation with which we approached the first patients. The patients were in pain and in a state of exquisite tenderness, so that light touch provoked a wince of pain. It might reasonably be predicted that electrical stimulation would produce an agonizing increase of pain. The actual result is that when the electrically produced tingling reaches the tender area, it becomes much less sensitive. This is one of the methods of stimulation we will now describe.

Transcutaneous Electrical Nerve Stimulation (TENS)

In this technique, large surface electrodes are taped to the skin to stimulate the underlying nerves that supply the painful area. Under the patient's control, the current is gradually increased until a tingling is felt. The stimulus is provided by a small, hand-held box, and the patient is in complete control after an initial training period. This technique is widely used in the United States and Europe for localized pains, for postoperative pain, and during labor.

Implanted Electrode Nerve Stimulation

In cases (which are quite rare) when the painful area is too extensive and the nerves cannot be reached from surface electrodes, electrodes can be implanted during surgical exposure of the nerves. The surgeon attaches these electrodes to a small radio receiver buried under the skin. The patient operates a hand-held radio transmitter, which stimulates the nerves as in TENS.

Dorsal Column Stimulation

Large-diameter peripheral nerve fibers, on entering the spinal cord, send out a branch that runs the entire length of the cord until it enters the skull, where nuclei are located. Therefore, gentle stimulation on the surface of the spinal cord produces a generalized tingling in the entire body below where the electrodes are placed. Electrodes to carry out this stimulation can easily be placed on the spinal cord by the technique used to insert a catheter for spinal-block anesthesia. Once again, the electrodes are connected to a radio receiver and the patient controls the transmitter when the pain increases. This is used particularly when there is injury to the spinal cord, as in paraplegia and in multiple sclerosis.

Vibration

Many of the large fibers can be driven into continuous activity by light mechanical vibrators powered by electricity. They are not so effective as the electrodes, but they are in common use because they are so simple. People with arthritis or muscle strains often find that they can achieve relief by this method.

Do-It-Yourself Stimulation

By this, we simply mean rubbing, licking, scratching, or light massage. Obviously, people and animals in pain have been doing this forever. All that is new is an understanding of the effect on the nerves, which works by exactly the same mechanism as electrical stimulation, though of course less intensively and consistently.

The simplest of these stimulation techniques are so safe that they can be used at home with freely purchased equipment. In the more elaborate methods of stimulation, the patient needs an introduction to the method by skilled hospital professionals, who can later turn the control over to the patient.

Stimulation therapies, especially TENS, are widely used in the treatment of acute pains associated with sporting injuries, surgical operations, childbirth, and angina pectoris. They are also useful for some chronic pains, including peripheral nerve disorders, spinal cord damage, cancer pains, muscle pains, and arthritis. They are not appropriate for extensive deafferentation pain syndromes, pains of spinal cord or thalamic origin, visceral pains, headaches, or pains whose source is psychogenic.

There is clearly a placebo component in stimulation, but tests have shown that the real effect of TENS is three times greater than the placebo effect. With paraplegics, who cannot feel pain in paralyzed parts of the body, TENS is helpful by reducing overactive reflexes. Even when a patient is anesthetized, TENS can reduce the amount of anesthetic needed to maintain the anesthesia.

Generally, stimulation therapy reduces the pain and makes it more bearable but does not eliminate it. As with most other therapies, the effect tends to fade after a few months. This does not mean that the disease is getting worse, though the patient may think so. Probably, the nervous system has an ability to counteract any treatment that interferes with its functioning, and unfortunately this includes the function of producing pain.

Folk Medicine

"Folk medicine" is a phrase that should not be used—and certainly we do not intend to use it—in a contemptuous or dismissive manner. It simply refers to remedies that have been traditionally applied by ordinary people without justification by an analytical theory. It is foolish to reject a therapy because its rationale is not understood by those using it; the relevant question is whether it does any good. We can reasonably think that the explanation popularly or traditionally believed (for instance, that a devil is driven out of the sufferer) is absurd, and yet allow value to the treatment.

What is certain is that people have been treating pain for a much longer span of history than they have been able to treat most diseases. In fact, it is impossible to imagine any society, however primitive, in which ways of alleviating pain were not developed. Most folk remedies for pain, as we see when we observe and describe them, are actually stimulation therapies. Long before electricity was mastered, heat treatments were in use all over the world in the form of hot baths, saunas, and heated dressings or poultices. Cooling by cold water or ice also produces its effect by generating nerve impulses from the skin. Herbal embrocations work by producing a reddening of the skin and a feeling of warmth. At the present level of civilization, we can still learn from folk medicine and adapt and improve on what is effective in it.

Acupuncture

Acupuncture originated in China and was first described in a medical treatise written around 1000 BC Small needles, generally made of steel, are inserted into the body at specified points. Traditional charts of the body indicate 365 points, situated on one or another of 12 lines known as meridians.

The philosophical rationale for this procedure is that health depends on a correct balance between the two human principles—the *yin*, or feminine, and the *yang*, or masculine. Excessive *yin* leads to tiredness and depression, while excessive *yang* leads to anxiety and tension. According to the symptoms reported (for example, headache or indigestion), the acupuncturist can discern where the imbalance arose and insert the needles suitably. Each acupuncture point is related to a specific organ, though in a literal sense it may be nowhere near that organ.

Acupuncture has been alternatively discovered and forgotten by the West. The first vogue was in the seventeenth century, when there was much admiration for Chinese wisdom. Another vogue came when French colonialists encountered it in Indochina (Balzac in 1829 made a joking reference to acupuncture). Weir Mitchell, describing the painful effects of wounds in the American Civil War, stated that "the Chinese needling does not reduce the pain." Within China, acupuncture was given high status under the rule of Mao Zedong, as it fitted into his doctrine that China should rely on her own resources and eschew imported models. In the 1970s, as Western contacts with China multiplied following President Nixon's visit, acupuncture was hailed as an exciting novelty by the American and

European public. However, after the death of Mao, the Chinese themselves laid less stress on its benefits. This history suggests that the effectiveness of acupuncture depends, at least to some extent, on socially induced belief.

When reports of acupuncture reached the West in recent times, excitement was evoked mainly by its use as an anesthetic in operations. There was something astonishing in the spectacle of a patient undergoing major surgery, not even oblivious to the outer world, as would be the case under hypnosis, but chatting about the news and the weather. Fuller knowledge, however, modified the excitement. It appears that anesthesia through acupuncture is feasible only when the patient is fully responsive to it (as with deep hypnosis), that a preliminary training course is necessary, and that the anesthesia is usually supplemented by pain-killing drugs. However, the Chinese had never valued acupuncture primarily for its anesthetic use, but rather as a therapy for a wide variety of afflictions, including obesity, malaria, dysentery, anxiety, depression, insomnia, neuralgia, and rheumatic and lumbar complaints—and in particular to relieve pain.

Acupuncturists vary considerably in the techniques they employ, and there have been systematic trials to evaluate the differences. Some make only a superficial penetration, while others probe deeply into muscle fascia and the periosteum. Once the needle is in place, some leave it stationary, but others maintain a steady movement, often aided by attaching it to a voltage source. Some patients feel little more than a series of pinpricks (or rather needle pricks), while others feel acute pain to the limit of tolerance.

Perhaps the most important distinction is this: some acupuncturists needle tender points related to a specific pain, whereas others needle the "classical points" all over the body. Fibromyalgia is a common condition characterized by tender points within muscle tissue, which evoke a sharp, radiating stab of pain if gently pressed. No one understands exactly what these trigger points are, but there is no doubt that they are real

and are often associated with distant referred pains and difficulty in movement. There is also no doubt that if a needle is
pushed into such a point, or if a local anesthetic is injected,
there is at least a temporary reduction in tenderness or pain.
The tender points are not scattered at random over the body, but
occur in predictable places. Many of them coincide with points
on the traditional acupuncture map designated as effective for
pain, so it may well be that successful acupuncture treatment is
identical with stimulation of tender points carried out by doctors who had never heard of acupuncture. Furthermore, since
pains of deep origin tend to present the appearance of pains
referred to distant areas of the same segment, stimulation
anywhere in that segment inhibits the perception of pain.

Skepticism in the Western medical world was evoked
mainly by the fact that the points and meridians did not consist
of observable bodily structures, and indeed had no apparent
reality. But comparison between the meridian chart and the
nervous system showed that many of the points were situated
close to the paths of peripheral nerves. In any case, pain was
reduced even when needles were inserted at what, according to
the chart, was the wrong place. This enabled Western doctors
(much to their relief) to reach an explanation of acupuncture in
their own terms, namely, that it works by stimulating pain-
inhibiting mechanisms in the central nervous system. The
stimulation itself, and its intensity, seem to be more important
than the location where it is initiated.

One of the authors (P.D.W.) was invited to investigate
acupuncture in China and observed surgical operations carried
out under acupuncture. There was no doubt of the reality of
this startling phenomenon, but there were strong clues to the
mechanism. It was never used on patients without their willing
cooperation and previous familiarization. At a large hospital
staffed by enthusiasts for acupuncture, it was admitted that
this ruled out 90% of operations—that is, emergency operations, procedures on children and old people unresponsive to
training, and abdominal operations. In other words, we were

witnessing an individual cognitive phenomenon, not a general property of the human body, as would be the case with an ordinary anesthetic. Out of 30 operations observed, large doses of strong narcotics and local anesthetics were used in addition to acupuncture in 28 cases; two patients, however, calmly underwent major surgery under acupuncture alone. This was evidence of the reality of the phenomenon, but also of its rarity.

Two of the cases provided further clues. One patient, to the astonishment of the Western visitors, showed no sign of pain when a major artery in the leg was exposed by dissection even before the acupuncture started. One could only conclude that her immunity to pain stemmed from confident expectation and verbal suggestion. Another patient suddenly emerged from his pain-free state and uttered horrifying screams at the end of the operation. Apparently, the surgeon had introduced a tube in the chest wall, which had not been explained to the patient during his training. Both these incidents are reminiscent of things that happen with patients under hypnosis.

The conclusion is that acupuncture works through two quite different effects. One is the needling of the tender points in the area of pain; the other is suggestion. Unfortunately, if one remarks on the presence of the latter, as we do here, one is often accused of disbelieving in the former. Dedicated adherents of a given theory—whether this is a Western theory expressed in scientific terms or the Chinese yin and yang system—tend to get very annoyed if it is argued that faith in the theory is a factor in the effectiveness of the therapy. In such attitudes, we can detect the persistence of the old dualistic outlook, which maintained that what happens physically or literally is real, while what happens in the mind is unreal.

But the importance of suggestion enables us to understand why acupuncture has been alternately in high and low esteem in the West, and for that matter in China too. In order to be acceptable and effective, the suggestion "You will not feel pain" must be made by a credible person—that is, a person respected for reasons of class, social status, authority, or presumed knowledge and wisdom. At a certain time and place, acupuncturists may be regarded as quacks or tricksters. (At other times and places, that view may be taken of orthodox medical practitioners.) To recognize this, however, is not to allege that the good effects of acupuncture, or of any other kind of alternative medicine, are anything other than valid and welcome. Patients who wish to try such a therapy should always be encouraged to do so. If it fails to help them, they are no worse off except that they may feel sad and discouraged. If it does help them, a victory has been achieved. (One caution: the patient should first satisfy himself that the diagnosis was correct.)

Physiotherapy: Heat and Cold

A traditional form of therapy, going back to the beginnings of medicine, is the use of heat and cold for the relief of pain, as well as for relaxation, refreshment, and recovery from weariness. A Roman legionary post is immediately identified when archaeologists discover hot and cold bathhouses, and there have been similar findings in Scandinavia, Russia, Japan, and American-Indian settlements. Nowadays, heat treatment localized to a given part of the body can be administered in two ways. Lamps, heating pads, poultices, and wax baths are methods of superficial treatment; ultrasound and short-wave microwave therapy are methods of deep heat treatment.

The effect of superficial heat treatment can be explained only as stimulation of fibers in the skin, because the body's homeostatic mechanisms prevent any rise in deep temperature. The skin stimulation sends in a sensory volley that produces a relaxation of underlying muscle. If the temperature rises to a noxious level, there is a counterirritant effect. As T. S. Eliot noted:

> Here comes the nurse with a red-hot poultice,
> Slaps it on and takes no notice.

The heating of deep body structures by ultrasound or microwave has the added advantage of a placebo effect. Elaborate shiny machinery with dials and flashing lights, manipulated by a sympathetic person in a white coat, can hardly fail to be impressive. A recent study of the effect of ultrasound in reducing swelling and pain after the extraction of wisdom teeth showed that it made no difference whether the machine was turned on or not, provided that both therapist and patient believed that something was happening. But heat undoubtedly produces reflex effects on muscle and blood vessels as well as direct local effects. There is good evidence that these can confer at least temporary relief from pain, so long as they do not exaggerate ongoing inflammatory reactions, which can make the pain worse by increasing swelling.

Similarly, the effect and mechanism of cold treatment depend on intensity and duration. Ice cubes are obviously painful when first applied and are a classic example of the counterirritation effect—not fighting fire with fire, but fighting fire with ice. More gentle cooling has a good local anti-inflammatory effect by constricting blood vessels and thus reducing swelling. It also changes the afferent sensory signals, and these in turn produce central effects and changes in reflex muscle contraction and in circulation. A common example of cooling as a reflex stimulus is the use of pain-relieving sprays. Often used in sports injuries, the "magic spray" has an immediate effect, which also lasts much longer than the superficial cooling of the skin.

In ancient and modern times, judicious use of heating and cooling, or an alternation of the two, is a well-cultivated art and a sound remedy for painful muscle contraction. This therapy is harmless, it is effective, and it is based on cooperation between patient and therapist, altogether, a good idea.

Massage

The antiquity of this therapy is borne out by the history of a cognate set of verbs: *makeh*, to stroke or press, in Sanskrit; *massein*, to knead, in Greek; *mass*, to touch, in Arabic; *mashesh*, to feel or touch, in Hebrew. Like heat therapy, relief of pain through touch at the right places and in the right rhythm has been practiced by unknown healers and ordinary people throughout human history. The orthodox medical establishment has generally been dismissive or hostile, and even today practitioners of manipulation and massage work in a half-recognized limbo. This is regrettable, for people in need of help have difficulty making a valid choice.

Massage in all its forms consists of local stimulation of nerves in soft tissue without moving the joints. Light stroking, clearly, affects only the skin. Deep stroking is supposed to free deep adhesions as well as having a stimulating effect, and it results in a feeling of warmth and a reddening of the skin. Kneading involves firm lifting, squeezing, and pushing of skin, subcutaneous tissue, and muscles. Friction massage and deep massage aim at (presumed) scars, adhesions, and trapped tendons. There is often an element of ritual in the treatment; percussion, clapping, and pummeling with rapid blows are in vogue at a Kikuyu village well or a Japanese military parade ground, just as in the more sophisticated ambience of spas and health farms. The placebo effect is obvious, as are the possibilities of enjoyment. Not too surprisingly, "massage parlor," "bathhouse," and "sauna" have become suspect terms, or sometimes recognized euphemisms for "brothel." It is arguable, however, that the connection is logical, and that the up-market prostitute in Tokyo or Bangkok, who provides her customer with a hot bath and an hour of massage as a preliminary to the final service, is functioning as a therapist too. There is no rigid dividing line, after all, between feeling good and being in good health.

Movement of the Joints and Muscles

Mobilization and stretching, as the words imply, aim at a progressive increase of the range over which joints can be comfortably moved. The methods vary from short, sharp jerks to rapid oscillations of gradually increasing amplitude. The idea is to stretch the ligaments and joint capsules so that a movement that the patient found difficult and painful becomes pain-free.

This therapy merges into the forcible manipulation of "locked" joints. It is possible to carry out an extreme manipulation when the patient is under general anesthesia. More commonly, after careful positioning of the patient on a special table, the manipulator wrenches joints in the desired direction, sometimes with the aid of forcible traction with adjustable block and tackle. These maneuvers are particularly directed at the vertebrae. It has yet to be proved that the application of force brings about specific vertebral movements. But, in this field as in others, the perceived benefit of the treatment matters more than the theory.

Massage (as distinct from manipulation) has never been subjected to a serious controlled trial. This is a pity, for the huge variety of techniques cannot all be equally effective for every condition and for each individual. A person who set out to try them all would need to be rich in both money and time.

Exercise

The intuitive message associated with pain is "Don't move." For this, there is a sound biological reason. When tissue is damaged and is in the process of repair, it makes sense to keep the damaged part as stationary as possible so that the cells that move into the area of injury can establish their proper contacts and work toward the best possible reconstruction. When we wish to repair a fracture, an artificial splinting with plaster is added to the body's own efforts to stabilize the two ends of the broken bone. If these are aligned and held stable, the bone can knit by exchanging cells across the gap, laying down new bone, and reestablishing continuity.

However, there are limits to this rule of immobility. Joints that are not moved tend to seize up because of the overgrowth of connective tissue. Lack of movement also leads to gradual atrophy of the muscles, and the final outcome can be the spindly limbs of people who have been held still for excessive periods. To avert these dangers, aided movement and then graded active exercise are necessary.

When injury occurs, muscles contract, first to withdraw the damaged area from further danger and then to hold it in a steady state. The muscle contraction plays some part in generating the pain, so it is desirable to make efforts to stop this contraction if the pain continues beyond its useful period. One of the most effective ways of doing this is through relaxation exercises, which take advantage of the subtle interplay between various components of the motor nervous system. For example, to take a step forward you must straighten your knee. So long as you hold it straight, the muscles used in bending it are under positive order to relax. By doing this, you can overcome pathological activity, not by brute force, but by making use of turnoff signals that already exist. Physiotherapists have become very skillful at teaching people how to do such exercises.

Another aspect of motor movement is surprising. When a voluntary movement is made, we might expect the brain to maximize the sensitivity of the part to be moved. But the opposite happens; movement is accompanied by a marked decrease of sensitivity. This phenomenon can be put to practical use. Suppose that a patient with a crippling acute attack of low back pain is lying in bed in agony. Every movement exaggerates the pain. Both the patient and the treatment team are naturally impelled to maintain immobility in order to minimize the pain and hold this position as long as necessary—days, weeks, or months—until the pain dies down. But therapists nowadays are coming to favor the idea of getting the patient moving, despite the reluctance of patients themselves and the objections of physiotherapists, who have been taught never to produce pain. Movement does work, for a logical reason. Patients who move to the limit of their tolerance (and indeed healthy people in training for some athletic purpose) find that the level of this tolerance steadily rises. As they embark on more movement, they prevent the stiffness and weakness caused by inactivity. More essentially still, the period of helpless domination by pain is shortened. The morale of the patient rises with the return of activity, even if it is only tottering to the bathroom. The patient who remains immobile is submitting to an arbitrary limit set by authority; the patient who attempts movement is exploring and enlarging his own capacities. Thus, exercise therapy aims to reestablish personal control over pain.

As we have seen, surgery designed to cut pain transmitters is decreasing, because the good effects are short-lived and less destructive methods have become available. Similarly, the use of surgery to relieve pressure is under critical examination. Instead of cutting tissue, there is now a vigorous exploration of stimulation, which helps the nervous system to regain its own normal pain-free state. While new methods of electrical stimulation are being added, there is a growing respect and understanding for the traditional methods, which use heat, cold, or pressure to aid people in pain.

10

Belief-and-Attitude Therapies

We shall now describe therapies that rely for their effectiveness on the patient's belief that they can be of help and on a positive attitude. A central theme of this book is that mind and body should be understood as an integrated whole. Therapy based on this assumption is sometimes called "holistic medicine," but this simply means medicine that takes all relevant factors into account—or, still more simply, good medicine. Doctors and patients should support any procedure that has a clear prospect of success, without first requiring a rationale and without worrying because a placebo factor may be involved. In our opinion, organizations that pay for medical treatment—such as the National Health Service in Britain, Medicare in the United States, and private insurance companies—should take this attitude too.

If we accept this view, we cannot agree with the classical theory that psychotherapy for pain becomes relevant only when medicine and surgery have failed. The doctrine of mind over matter, popular with certain macho types who like to boast of the strength of their own minds, is ignorant in its essence and cruel in its callousness toward people in pain. It is sad indeed to observe the bewilderment of these macho characters when they themselves are in severe pain.

Every pain in every individual is affected by that person's attitude, mood, and understanding. Here, we are not discussing those rare and unfortunate people whose thought processes, speech, and behavior are so grossly disturbed that they are really insane. Such people may express their delusions and hallucinations in terms of pain. Psychiatrists in charge of these patients must remain alert to the possibility that they may be suffering from treatable diseases in addition to their mental disturbance. Turning to the great majority of human beings who use comprehensible language, we will start with a topic that is at the heart of the entire subject.

PLACEBO THERAPY

This subject is extremely unpopular for two reasons. Therapists, whether orthodox or unorthodox, operate on a theory that explains why their therapy works. They are therefore disturbed and angry if it is suggested that some or all of their patients are responding to a belief in the theory rather than to the mechanism on which the theory is based. They take such a suggestion as a personal attack on them and their ideas. The fact is that no therapy is 100% successful and that a percentage of successes are placebo responses. Furthermore, it is not a question of which effects are "real" and which are due to placebos, because the real effects contain a placebo component. Patients dislike mention of the placebo response because they fear that if they are shown to respond, it will signify that their pain was imaginary in the first place. These patients are victims of the strict application of dualistic thinking, in which a pain is either appropriate to an injury or is an invention of the mind. They are then persuaded that a placebo response means that the pain was a hallucination. All this antipathy and anger is unfortunate because it submerges a marvelous common phenomenon which should be exploited for the benefit of patients, rather than dismissed as a diversion from proper treatment.

The detailed observation of a placebo response is remarkable. If a cancer patient has been receiving regular narcotics for his pain, the secret substitution of a blank dose, unknown to him or the nurse, is followed by pain relief. The time course of onset and duration of analgesia precisely mimics those which occurred when the narcotic was given. Moreover, the response is not just verbal. There is a drop of heart rate, breathing is easier, and, a side effect of which the patient is completely unaware, pupil constriction also occurs. In other words, the placebo response includes the full range of expected and unexpected signs and symptoms. It is unrelated to the intensity of the pain. A crucial aspect of the placebo response is that if the blank dose is repeated again and again, the effect fades.

Placebos are not limited to pain but have marked effects on swelling, appetite, sleep, and motion sickness, and probably on many conditions that have not been tested. Nor are they limited to human beings. Rats show a spectacular example of one-trial learning related to their skill in avoiding poisoned bait. If a rat is once injected with a noxious substance in a definite location, its sickness behavior on that occasion will be repeated if the rat is given a saline injection in the same location 6 months later. There are even light-hearted experiments that the reader can try. If cups of decaffeinated instant coffee are secretly served in a random order with cups of normal instant coffee, a person who experiences finger tremor after drinking coffee will experience the same tremor after drinking a cup of decaffeinated.

The placebo is treated as an annoying intrusion, which confuses the proper analysis of "true" actions. When a new drug is invented, it is required by law that its action must be shown to be superior to that of a placebo. This is done by a double-blind trial in which a blank tablet indistinguishable from the real thing is given. For every analgesic, a marked percentage of patients and normal volunteers respond identically to the two tablets. This need to "fool" the subject and the observer so that they cannot distinguish between the blank and the true treatment places a severe restriction on this method of testing. Take, for example, a test of acupuncture. How are you to fool patient and therapist with the psychological equivalent of a needle without using a needle? In practice, no such tests can be devised; the best that can be done is to compare the effects of two overtly different treatments. These tests do not probe what may be an intense faith or belief in the value of acupuncture, because everyone knows that acupuncture has not been used in the matching trial.

If a treatment such as acupuncture is difficult to test, the problems are multiplied when we consider surgery. A book by Dr. Bernard Finneson (20) includes the following startling sentences: "Probably surgery has the most potent placebo effect that can be exercised in medicine. The detailed preliminaries, the rendering unconscious via anesthesia and the removal or manipulation of vital organs within the body all create an almost mystic and profound emotional effect on the patient." Having made this statement, the author goes on to describe any number of surgical operations without once evaluating this effect. It would clearly be completely unethical to subject a patient to a fake operation, which would necessarily involve some danger, in order to test the validity of the procedure. Doctors are required by their own conscience and by law never to touch a patient unless their action is intended to help that specific patient. This prohibition of the use of humans as sacrificial guinea pigs thereby prohibits testing of complex treatments and leaves surgeon and patient dependent on belief and trust.

Nevertheless, unwitting trials occur on occasions. It sometimes happens during surgery that the operation must stop because of blood pressure collapse. There are a number of reports in medical literature of patients who do not know that the intended operation was not carried out, but experience an excellent result. The largest unwitting placebo trial in surgery occurred before the days of coronary bypass surgery. It was known that angina and heart trouble were associated with an inadequate blood supply to heart muscle, and it seemed reasonable to divert arteries from the chest wall and implant them in heart muscle. When this was done, many patients felt better, had less pain, and moved more easily. Only when vascular X-rays improved did it become apparent that this operation in fact made absolutely no difference to the blood supply of the heart. The operation was replaced by bypass surgery, which does improve circulation.

We should try to move away from the negative attitude to placebos, which regards them as irritating intrusions on real effects. For this, we need to demystify. A placebo is not a mere object, but a procedure finely tuned to the society in which the subject lives. In the West, there is an ascending scale of power of analgesic placebos as follows: white round tablet, least effective; then shaped tablets, colored tablets, and capsules; then intramuscular injections; and, most effective, intravenous injections. Clearly, this hierarchy reflects the reputation of the procedures and must have been learned. Reputations for effectiveness will differ between individuals and societies. The need to learn is shown by the fact that young children do not respond to placebo medicines; they have other magic recipes, such as "mother kissing it better." The learning process has recently been studied by an imaginative group of psychologists at La Trobe University in Australia (68). They played innocent tricks on their volunteer subjects, who were given painful stimuli to the forearm. Then a bland cream was put on the arm, which they were told had anesthetic properties. Next, the experimenters secretly turned down the strength of the painful stimulus, thereby imitating the expected action of the cream. A few trials like this convinced the subjects that the cream was wonderful. After this training, the cream had a powerful placebo effect when the stimulus was not turned down and even when other painful stimuli were given.

This phenomenon is reminiscent of the conditioning described by Pavlov. A dog salivates when hearing a bell that has become associated with food. Appropriate responses occur when associated stimuli are given even in the absence of the unconditioned stimulus. There is a second, very important similarity with conditioned responses. If the bell rings repeatedly but no food appears, the conditioned response fades unless food is given at least occasionally. That is unfortunately the case when placebos have to be repeated. Yet another similarity is that conditioned stimuli evoke the full pattern of conscious and unconscious responses, not just verbal statements.

We can now ask whether the placebo effect is a special isolated phenomenon, or whether it relates to other aspects of pain. In discussing the dramatic occurrence of emergency analgesia (injury without pain), we concluded that pain occurs by permission of the brain when the brain decides that pain is biologically relevant. If the past experience of the brain has taught it that certain procedures are followed by relief of pain, the brain withdraws permission to feel pain and proceeds with some other, more pleasant form of behavior. This brain process can include prediction, a necessary attribute of complex brains, which do not await the definite arrival of an expected trigger stimulus before initiating what will become appropriate behavior. The athlete on the starting block has initiated not just awareness and attention, but the full complex of increased heart rate, blood flow, mobilized blood sugar, and so on long before the starter's pistol actually fires. We have seen repeatedly that the brain possesses machinery to select appropriate behavior not just in relation to single moment-by-moment events, but also in relation to the entire ensemble of present events with knowledge from the past and with predictions for the future. The brain can be "fooled" into selecting an apparently appropriate form of behavior by presenting it with a fraction of the relevant stimuli, the placebo. Can we move from fooling the brain to using that same mechanism in a more rational way? You can only fool some of the brain some of the time. Since the brain is certainly smart enough to detect fooling, the placebo effect fades. Hence, we need ways to help the brain to adopt this strategy honestly and rationally.

PSYCHOTHERAPY

Depression, anxiety, stress, tension, and pain are unholy devils, which chase each other round in a circular dance. There is little point in selecting one member of the gruesome corps de ballet and blaming it for the choreography. The patient is not trapped alone in this swirl but is accompanied by friends, relatives, and therapists; each makes a contribution for better or worse. No matter what may be the cause of the pain, it is intensified by anxiety, depression, stress, and tension. It is better when the victim is at ease and distracted. There are unfriendly friends who will say, "He can't be in real pain. I saw him laughing while playing cards." Such statements are the uncharitable consequence of dualistic thinking in which "real" pain must be unaffected by the workings of the mind.

Anxiety could obviously play a role in two different ways, which are not exclusive. The anxiety and the pain could be interlocked and compounded. The facial expressions of pain and anxiety are hard to tell apart. Even the words are mixed up. "She is a real pain" means "she irritates me." Studies of physiological variables such as heart rate, tremor, and sweating do not differentiate between anxiety and pain. It is possible that pain interacts only with that anxiety which is specifically related to the pain. On the other hand, a person can have plenty of reasons to be anxious about matters that have nothing to do with pain itself. For example, an impending visit to the dentist can certainly be a source of rising anxiety because of the anticipated pain. Alternatively or additionally, it can be a source of anxiety because of the formidable bill. Both types of anxiety increase the pain.

There have been many investigations related to this rather important point, which again shows that pain is not an isolated mechanism but is woven into the integrated human experience. A group of 64 students volunteered for a pain tolerance test and were paid 10 dollars for their trouble (15). Each had gradually rising pressure applied to a finger and rated their pain levels and stress while various physiological measures were taken. They could call quits whenever it became intolerable. One group was made anxious about the pain test by being told that prolonged exposure was dangerous (which it was not). Another group was made generally anxious by being told that they would soon have an interview to test their intelligence and personality. Both the anxious groups showed similar increased pain ratings, stress intensity ratings, and heart rate increases. Interestingly, none of the groups differed in their actual tolerance of pain, but the anxious ones did show stronger overt responses to pain and stress.

In practice, there is every reason to use all possible methods to decrease anxiety in people in pain. This book is itself such an attempt with its implication that knowledge, understanding, and control are prerequisites for rational anxiety reduction. Beyond this, pain may be so bad that there is a need for professional intervention. The accident victim or the war casualty can be in as much trouble with terror as with pain of injury. The cancer patient may be more anxious about the expectation of rising pain than about death itself.

Depression, with its accompanying feelings of helplessness and grief, intertwines with pain in the same way as anxiety. Sickness and pain are depressing. Depression for any reason or for no reason may be experienced as pain. Depression or anxiety may occur for no obvious reason, or as a reaction to death, divorce, unemployment, or any of the misery-making events that afflict us. Recently, an unselected group of 32 men who had had low back pain for more than 6 months was studied in San Diego (3). Fifteen of them were overtly depressed while the other seventeen were not depressed, though the amount of pain and physical impairment was about the same in both groups. This tells us two things. It is evident that depression is very prevalent among back pain sufferers, but on the other hand, some people have back pain even though they are not depressed. Next, the two groups and also 19 men who were not in pain were questioned about their recent experience of events likely to distress and depress them. The depressed group had a significantly larger number of such events than the other two groups. Furthermore, all the depressed patients were found to be under continuing stress, while similar degrees of stress were found in only 47% of the men in the other two groups. Stress and depression do not necessarily go with chronic back pain, but they are associated in a large number of cases.

A striking report has appeared on amputees who were peasants in the Uttar Pradesh state in India. Depression was invariable and intense. A Western reader soon realizes that he does not know what it means, even in practical terms of survival, to be an amputee in this poverty-stricken part of the world. Further, the largest cause of amputation was that an arm had been chopped off by a band of robbers. Such amputees share the common experience of all amputees, but with an additional misery, which is difficult to imagine.

Depression may be so serious that professional help is needed in the form of counseling, either one to one or in group sessions. Antidepressant medicines may also be prescribed. As we have pointed out, these drugs have a fortunate side effect in addition to their antidepressant action. They act by building up the concentration in the brain of compounds such as serotonin. Serotonin is involved in one of the inhibitory mechanisms that operate the gate control. Therefore, these tricyclic antidepressants have an analgesic effect in addition to the action for which they were designed.

We have written repeatedly in this book that we deplore the crude dualism that separates mind from body and sensation from perception. That does not mean that the experience of pain is single and indivisible. For example, some pains are sickening. That refers to the affective response to the pain and is different from the pain. Beyond this, there are the cognitive components, which come from thinking about the pain and the injury. For example, we described a young woman with a leg blown off but not yet in pain. With tears streaming down her face, she said, "Who is going to marry me now?" She was thinking and making a cognitive prediction (which fortunately turned out to be wrong). These sensory, affective, and cognitive components also form an interactive interlocking system. Thinking about the meaning of an event is natural and appropriate. However, some of us come to inappropriate and obsessional conclusions about meanings. That is neurotic thinking.

There are two forms of neurosis that involve pain. The hypochondriac has four lifelong characteristics. He has a fear of illness. In itself, such a fear is rational and understandable. It is a characteristic of neurosis that every thought, feeling, and action is understandable, but the appropriateness is in question. It may be appropriate for some people to fear disease more than others. If someone has a strong family history of diabetes, he may reasonably fear diabetes more than the rest of us and be alert for early minor signs. However, the fears of a hypochondriac go far beyond those of most of us who take acceptable risks in our daily lives. Fears restrict the freedom of the fearful and intrude on the lives of others. A hypochondriac is not free to share a cup of tea with a friend for fear of caffeine, polluted water, cholesterol in the milk, and an inadequately washed cup. If the friend persists in the offer, he must change his style of brewing tea.

The second characteristic of hypochondriacs is a preoccupation with body signs and symptoms. If anyone scans his body from top to toe for unusual feelings, he is sure to detect something odd. If attention is fearfully locked on to an itch, a twinge, a numbness, an ache, it is sure to grow and persist. We are a gallery of signs and symptoms available for introspection and inspection. The feces have a frequency, shape, consistency, color, and smell of sufficient variability to occupy a connoisseur of such matters full time. Once an abnormal symptom has been detected, it is an easy step to the next characteristic of the hypochondriac, which is a conviction that he has a disease. The word comes from *hypo*, meaning below, and *chondria*, the ribs. It originates from the common belief in some cultures that the liver is a delicate organ from which all manner of complaints arise, hence our words "liverish" and "melancholia," meaning "black bile." The fourth characteristic of the hypochondriac is that he is unable to accept reassurance. If a medical test produces a finding of normality, the hypochondriac insists that the doctor who carried it out is incompetent. Obsessive phobias are sad, disruptive, and dangerous for the patient. Self-imposed inactivity has its dangers. The intercurrence of treatable disease is missed or dismissed by those who have heard the hypochondriac "cry wolf" too often. Worst of all, these miserable obsessive phobias are extremely resistant to all forms of psychotherapy.

A second type of neurotic behavior is called a conversion disorder. These people do not have a life history of fears and preoccupations with health and disease. They exhibit a body state such as blindness or paralysis or pain, for which no medical cause can be discovered. In the nineteenth century such a condition was called hysteria. The word was dropped for two reasons. Its origin was *hysteros*, Greek for the womb (hence, hysterectomy, meaning to cut out the womb). The implication was that it was a disease of women, and hysteria in men was considered impossible. Second, the word is commonly associated with being wildly out of control, whereas these patients present their condition with a remarkably calm resignation, called *la belle indifférence* by the French neurologists who first spotted the condition. It was their work which led Sigmund Freud to concentrate on such people in his first classical cases.

The term "conversion disorder" means that these people have converted some general cognitive problem into a specific body problem. They are not overt simulators or lead-swingers who are imitating disease for their benefit. They have covertly transferred a paradoxical cognitive problem in which they are trapped into a body problem that attracts their attention and that of others. Clearly, they present a difficult problem of medical diagnosis. For example, they may have a small, diagnosable disease that has been amplified by hysterical overlay.

Even more difficult is the assumption that medical diagnosis is so good that it can detect any disease. We have written about the 70% of low back pain sufferers in whom no explanatory lesion can be discovered. Are we therefore to label these millions as suffering some modern epidemic of hysteria? Some classical physicians and surgeons do just that. We prefer the explanation that the vast majority suffer from the induced hyperexcitability of spinal cord circuitry that we have described, while admitting that a very small percentage are in a conversion disorder. These patients respond to skillful, patient, sympathetic psychotherapy, which converts the body solution back to a cognitive problem and then tackles it for what it is.

THERAPIES DIRECTED AT BEHAVIOR AND BELIEF

We have just described two forms of neurosis that can be so extreme that no one, except the patient, has difficulty in recognizing them. They lie at one end of a continuous spectrum, with the normal person at the other end. Moving along this spectrum from the neurotic or psychotic extreme, phrases such as "psychogenic pain disorder" and "idiopathic pain disorder" are used. Idiopathic pain means a complaint of pain without associated injury; we have already discussed this problem. Briefly, the problem remains that the pain might be an individual cognitive invention of the patient or it might be a poorly recognized disordered pattern of neural function. Whatever the answer, the individual's attitude, culture, knowledge, and experience will stamp an individual face on the pain. The individuality of each person's pain experience is the reason why everyone, patient and physician, has such difficulty in this intermediate zone in deciding whether the experience is predominantly a personal invention or whether it is predominantly forced on the victim by design faults inherent in all bodies. Because of this quandary, diagnosis and treatments vary with fashion and fad. To some at some times, back pains, migraines, and painful phantom limbs are all neuroses. To others, they are organic diseases.

Moving further along the spectrum toward normal, there is an inevitable and justified reaction to pain, which will include fear, anxiety, depression, seeking help, and searching for comfort. The therapeutic problem is whether this behavior is appropriate. "Appropriate" is a value in the mind of the observer. The patient may be labeled as making a terrible fuss over nothing or as irresponsibly neglecting something. Much of the advice given to the patient is directed at pushing him into the advisor's normal range of behavior. Obviously, this advice is an expression of well-meaning concern. While none of us get the answer right, some of us get it wildly wrong. Here there is a real need for psychological and psychiatric help for both patient and friends.

Behavior therapy is one method used to bring the balance of behaviors into an appropriate range. It is based on the principle that behavior is governed by its consequences. This extremely powerful and fundamental statement is at the center of intense contemporary controversy. The theory is that if a behavior results in reward, it is repeated and exaggerated. On the other hand, if a behavior is ignored or even punished, it dies out or does not develop.

Before setting out to readjust a patient's behavior, there are two essential prerequisites. The first is that the best possible diagnosis has been made so that there is no possibility of missing some other beneficial therapy that can proceed along with the psychotherapy. The second is that the best possible prognosis is available so that a realistic goal can be the aim. The reaction of Lazarus to the order that he should take up his bed and walk is not an example of behavior therapy. It is usual to start the therapy with the signing of an agreed contract between patient and therapist on the realistic goals that are believed to be achievable and desirable. An example of a goal would be to walk to the bathroom or the garden or the shops. A decrease of intake of mind-boggling drugs is a frequent goal. The patient is then subjected to a graded series of encouragements, rewards, and praises for each tiny move toward the goal and a corresponding discouragement for each failure. In this way an attempt is made to shape behavior. The desired end result is obviously reversible if the patient reverts to a situation that encourages a return to the starting point. When badly done, this type of therapy can lead to considerable antagonism in the patient who feels that he has, in effect, been ordered by an unsympathetic authority to stop complaining.

Cognitive therapy is based on a quite different school of thought from behavioral therapy. Here the idea starts from the mind and moves out to behavior, in contrast to the behaviorist belief that external reactions, the consequences of behavior, shape the setting of the mind. It therefore concentrates on teaching the patient ways of thinking by changing attention, by redefining the experience as a different sensation, by distraction, and so on. The aim is to help the patient change his own habits of thinking rather than to manipulate the external environment to enforce a new way of feeling. This places the emphasis on the patient as the active initiator of perception and as the person responsible for adaptive ways of thinking. After initial individual assessment, the individual may learn in a group, which is not an authoritarian drill but an efficient way for some individuals to explore themselves. The patients are given training exercises and homework in attention, distraction, coping, reassessment of sensory experience, self-assertion, and so on.

A special version of behavior therapy teaches *relaxation*. It may seem contradictory that movement and exercise should be encouraged in the same patients who are taught relaxation, but we must remember that is it impossible to relax when attention is riveted on pain. The problem is how to bring about a shift of attention, and the answer is sometimes given in terms of activity. "Why don't you do something instead of just sitting there?" is an age-old question, whether aimed at children, the old, depressed people, or people in pain. Attempts are also made to wrench attention away from pain by the chanting of mantras or the singing of hymns. This may work for some people, but inducing a state of relaxation is more likely to relieve obsessive concentration on pain. Relaxation therapy has the added benefit of relieving the abnormal muscle contraction provoked by injury.

Meditation may begin with relaxation, but goes far beyond the passivity implied by the word "relaxation" and proceeds into intense struggle. It has been used in all religions as a positive achievement; what is achieved is a rare and difficult state of awareness. The intensity of the effort required is well described in the second chapter of Aldous Huxley's *Grey Eminence*. Few people succeed in using meditation to this full extent.

HYPNOSIS

Hypnosis—the word derives from *hypnos*, Greek for sleep—can be described as a condition resembling sleep into which one person is plunged by the commanding influence of another person, the hypnotist. Opinions differ as to whether the hypnotized state is actually the same as sleep. People who are hypnotized do not generally close their eyes, unless on the order of the hypnotist, but they are oblivious of external events of which they would normally be conscious. For us, the importance of hypnosis is that it can render the subject immune to physical sensations such as extreme heat or cold, and hence to pain.

First explored by the pioneering Swiss physician Paracelsus (1490–1541), hypnotism attracted widespread attention in the early nineteenth century. It was often known either as mesmerism (after Friedrich Mesmer, a practitioner with a gift for dramatization) or as animal magnetism, from a theory that its working depended on magnetic forces. It was particularly welcomed because it could induce a state of anesthesia—an exciting prospect at a time when other anesthetics did not yet exist. James Esdaile, a British surgeon working in Calcutta, performed many major operations and amputations on patients who, deep in what Esdaile called "magnetic sleep," were free from pain.

From about 1840, the practice of hypnotism went into a decline, at least in Britain (it continued to progress and to be viewed with respect in France). One reason was that ether and chloroform offered a simple, quicker means of producing anesthesia. Also, hypnotism was discredited by its exploitation by showmen and charlatans, so that the conservative oligarchs of the medical world were able to stigmatize it as quackery. At least one leading London doctor was driven out of the profession because of his championship of hypnotism.

By the end of the century, however, hypnotism had become at least permissible. Doctors were using it for the relief of pain (to the degree that anyone at that time was interested in relieving pain) and in cases involving mental illness, insomnia, neuralgia, rheumatism, epilepsy, drug addiction, and even seasickness. Today, although prejudice against hypnotism is still not altogether extinct, its value is generally recognized, but in the sphere of psychiatry more than in other fields of medicine. All modern psychiatric hospitals employ hypnotism as a regular technique.

There is ample evidence that people in a hypnotized state can be given relief from various forms of severe pain, including phantom limb pain. Volunteers in experiments have submitted to being cut and burned and have reported that their sensations did not amount to anything definable as pain. Following in Esdaile's tradition, surgeons operate on patients under hypnosis. Yet the curious fact is that although hypnosis has been a well-known phenomenon for about two centuries, the exact mechanism in the nervous system and the brain is far from being thoroughly understood.

Observations and experiments have led to the conclusion that hypnosis works by excluding the anxiety that normally goes with pain. Richard Sternbach wrote, "When the attention or reaction are interfered with or diminished, the stimulus is perceived as a sensation devoid of pain" (60). Another researcher found that people under hypnosis felt no pain from electric shocks, although they did experience effects such as skin changes like anyone else. He deduced that "the essence of hypnosis is the subject's conviction of the truth of the hypnotist's suggestions."

Hypnosis has two significant limitations. One is that, almost invariably, its effects are temporary. There are few, if any, cases of a chronically painful condition being permanently banished by hypnotism. However, for reasons to be shortly explained, some lasting benefit does result.

The other limitation is that by no means everyone can be hypnotized. William MacDougall in 1910 asserted that "hypnosis can be induced in the great majority of normal persons" and quoted experienced hypnotists as claiming a 90% success rate, but these estimates are now regarded as overoptimistic. We now distinguish between deep hypnosis, capable of obliterating severe pain and effecting anesthesia for major operations, and lighter hypnosis, which reduces sensitivity to stimuli such as heat. Probably no more than 30% of people can be plunged into deep hypnosis, most of us are susceptible to hypnosis to varying degrees, and about 10% are totally resistant to it. One theory is that acutely anxious people—in other words, those in whom anxiety is a major component of the pain experience—are particularly responsive to hypnosis. Certainly, hypnosis belongs emphatically in the domain of therapies that rely on belief and attitude.

It should be added that the service of a hypnotist are not invariably necessary. Some people—thanks either to training and practice or to innate ability—are capable of achieving the same results by means of self-hypnosis (also called autosuggestion). Masters of self-hypnosis include, presumably, Indian yogis who walk on hot coals and the medieval Christian mystics who submitted themselves to mortification of the flesh. We marvel at reports of the calmness of martyrs burned at the stake, and of more modern martyrs—a Czech student protesting against the Russian occupation, a Buddhist monk protesting against American intervention in Vietnam, who died in a blaze of petrol. It seems possible that autosuggestion, stimulated by intense and resolute faith, enabled them not to feel the pain that would reduce the ordinary person to helpless screaming.

While all these forms of psychotherapy have aspects in common, each differs in the focus of its aim, and each must be tuned to the needs and capacities of the individual. There can be no strictly defined, ritualized performance of a single type of therapy. Indeed, there is good reason to apply several types simultaneously because they are likely to have additive effects. Pain clinics, which we shall describe in Chapter 11, are a good setting for psychotherapy in combination with other forms of treatment. They are an environment that discourages the flourishing of cults and encourages an open-minded exploration of every available technique.

Relaxation, meditation, hypnosis, exercises with a physiotherapist—and for that matter, sexual pleasure or playing chess—all have an effect on pain by bringing about a shift of attention. The problem is "what to do for encores," because no one can achieve these states of distraction forever. The intrusion of the real world—hunger, the call of nature, or the ringing of the phone—gives pain a chance to reassert itself. Fortunately, however, patients who benefit from distraction, relaxation, and exercise therapies do not revert to square one when the therapies finish. There are three reasons for this. First, therapies break into the self-perpetuating circle of anxiety and pain. Second, they induce an improved physical fitness and sense of well-being, hitherto prohibited by the inactivity imposed by pain. Finally, they build a sense of confidence; sufferers are given cause to feel that they have ways of coping. It has been shown in a number of these programs that, while the pain itself is unchanged, sufferers achieve a lifestyle of increased freedom. They are able to move better, experience more pleasures, and engage in more activities, thus escaping from the total domination of pain.

We have seen that known methods of fighting against pain are many, varied, and resourceful. Yet, to make the best use of these methods, two requirements are essential. There must be people—health professionals, patients, and others—capable of a resolute dedication to achieving everything that is possible. And there must be a well-designed organizational structure in which these efforts can be effectively maintained. We shall go on to describe what is currently being done in this sphere.

11

Fighting against Pain

As we have seen, significant and heartening advances in the treatment of pain have been made in recent decades. But, with the knowledge that has been accumulated, much more could be done than is being done at present. One very active and successful group is the World Health Organization's expert committee on cancer pain. However, the WHO's 1990 report (74), after describing the work of this group in encouraging terms, adds a section headed "Obstacles to Implementation." It is worth quoting in full:

> The greatest improvement in quality of life for cancer patients and their families could be effected by implementation of existing knowledge of pain and symptom control. In a number of countries, the situation has improved considerably over the past 20 years for reasons that include:
> —the development of palliative care centers;
> —a greater understanding of the use of analgesic drugs;
> —demands from patients and families for better symptom control;
> —a consensus that adequate symptom control and a good quality of life are particularly important in patients with advanced disease.
> Globally, however, palliative care is still a neglected area and several million cancer patients suffer needlessly every day as a

result. The major obstacles to the implementation of palliative care appear to be:

- —absence of national policies on cancer pain relief and other aspects of palliative care;
- —lack of education for health care workers, policy-makers, administrators and the general public;
- —concern that the medical use of morphine and related drugs will fuel the problem of drug abuse in the community and result in increased restrictions on prescribing and supply;
- —limitations on supply and distribution of the drugs needed for the relief of pain and other symptoms, particularly in developing countries;
- —restrictions imposed by the adoption of regional, district or hospital formularies, which do not contain sufficient drugs for the control of pain and other symptoms;
- —shortage of professional health care workers empowered to prescribe analgesics and other drugs;
- —lack of financial resources for research and development in palliative care.

With this caution in mind, we go on to describe just what is being done where the battle against pain is being effectively waged. We have several times mentioned Professor J. J. Bonica of Seattle as the pioneer of the modern study of pain. After early work in Tacoma he set up the world's first comprehensive pain clinic in Seattle's main hospital. The idea that pain is a problem in itself distinct from problems of disease, and that doctors should devote their time and energy to it—an idea challenging many deep-rooted prejudices—was revolutionary indeed in the 1960s, and the struggle for its acceptance is by no means over as we write in 1991. Yet the steady proliferation of pain clinics has proved that it was an idea whose time had come.

The basic and essential characteristic of the pain clinic is that it is multidisciplinary. It is staffed by a team of professionals who, in the past, would have worked in separate departments and merely referred patients from one to another. The benefits for patients are obvious; in favorable cases, they find their pain understood and treated far sooner than under the old system.

Doctors and other professionals benefit too; they are able to learn from one another, to discuss new therapies outside their own field of specialization, and to gain access more conveniently to comparative data on the relative effectiveness of one or another therapy. In particular, the multidisciplinary clinic, including psychologists and psychiatrists along with physicians and physiotherapists, bridges the traditional gulf between care of the body and care of the mind. It symbolizes, and also confirms and strengthens, our understanding of pain as a unitary human experience.

Pain clinics now exist in every large hospital in North America and most European countries. Naturally, some are better than others, and it can also be said that some are more multidisciplinary than others. It is easy to post the sign "Pain Clinic" on the door of a room in which the patient sees the same doctor who would have seen him anyway. There is also the danger (since there is no copyright in the name) of fashionable charlatans cashing in on the pain clinic idea. By and large, however, it is unquestionable that pain clinics are providing a service that was only a dream a generation ago.

A PAIN CLINIC AT WORK

Dr. Douglas Justins, a consultant anesthetist, presides over the pain clinic at St. Thomas's, a big teaching hospital in London. His team includes a physician with a specialty in virology (she is currently studying the pain associated with AIDS), a clinical psychologist, a psychiatrist, a physiotherapist, an acupuncturist, a social worker, and a nurse with special training in pain problems.

Becky is the first case of the morning. She is a bright, composed young woman whose life revolves around athletics;

she normally competes in the 6-mile run. She has a pain in her left knee, severe enough for her to wear a brace. The cause of the pain is unknown; Becky is sure that it didn't start through an accident, and there is no sign of injury. She has been examined by an orthopedic specialist who is said to know more about knees than anyone else in the country, if not the world, and he is baffled.

The treatment tried so far is blocking of sympathetic nerves by injections. Becky says that this does bring relief, but the relief is temporary. Justins tells her to use the leg as much as possible during periods of relief and try to recreate normal functioning—even run if she can manage it.

Les is a man of 50 who developed cancer of the stomach 3 years ago. He underwent an operation, which was successful. This year, however, his stomach has been giving him pain again. He's naturally worried that the cancer is recurring, but examination has produced no evidence that it is. "It's hard to understand," Les says. The pain is severe in the early morning, but "a dull pain, pretty tolerable" at other times. He has given up his job in local government and spends almost all of his time at home. He has been prescribed MST (a morphine compound, taken in tablets). Justins advises him to increase the dose when he feels severe pain—take as much as he thinks necessary. Discussing the case, the team agree that if Les can suppress the pain, he will stop worrying about it so much; we have an example of pain closely associated with anxiety. Because Les is using the drug purely for its effect on pain, not for psychedelic action, Justins doesn't think that addiction is a danger. The overriding consideration is that morphine is needed; without it, both the anxiety and the pain would escalate. On the other hand, it would have been quite wrong to prescribe morphine for Becky. She has the resources to help herself without it, and furthermore, the pain she experiences may well be a type of pain that does not respond to narcotics.

Ethel is the next patient. The team exchange smiles: "Ah yes, Ethel." She has been regular visitor for the last few years.

Ethel is an 82-year-old woman, soon to celebrate her diamond wedding anniversary. She is short and stocky and comes across as a perky Cockney character—strong-minded, definite in her opinions, determined not to be fooled or put off with the wrong answers.

Ethel's story goes back to 1982, when her general practitioner told that she had a growth that might be cancerous and sent her to St. Bartholemew's Hospital for an exploratory operation. There was in fact no cancer, and Ethel blames the doctor: "It was her fault, frightening me like that. Still, she's dead herself now," Ethel adds, not without satisfaction. Justins tells her firmly that the doctor acted correctly. A few days after coming out of the hospital, Ethel fell in the street. A few days after that, she bent down at home to pick up something she'd dropped and felt a sharp pain—"I felt my skin tearing"— followed by a discharge of blood from the vagina. She has suffered from perineal pain ever since. The persistence of this pain is puzzling, because the torn tissue should soon have healed. Changing her mind as she tells the story, Ethel sometimes blames her troubles on the unnecessary operation, sometimes on the fall in the street, sometimes on the incident at home.

She has had two dilatation and curettage operations at St. Thomas's, has consulted a urologist (privately), has been to an acupuncturist (also privately), and has been sent to a psychiatrist. The acupuncturist, who is Chinese, decided that Ethel's urinary channels were blocked. The psychiatrist prescribed electroshock for depression; Ethel says, "That was all a mistake, I'm never depressed." The pain won't go away, and she takes Mogadon in order to sleep. Now she has been sent back to the pain clinic by the neurology department. Jan, the virologist, who has joined the clinic recently and hasn't seen Ethel before, examines her, finds inflammation, and recommends an examination by the dermatology department. "I don't mind, I'll give them a try," Ethel says. Justins thinks she'll be back at the pain clinic, but that's how the system works; it is a matter of principle never to turn away anyone who is still in pain.

Frank, the next patient, is a man who has really had troubles. He has had four operations, three for stomach ulcers and one, as he puts it, for "repairing the plumbing." He has also had a heart attack, shingles, and neuralgia, and still suffers from psoriasis. He has intermittent pain in his chest or his stomach, which he describes as "like rubbing sandpaper inside my skin." Frank is 62, but looks at least 10 years older. He is a skinny, undersized man, with the sort of physique that was more common in the 1930s than now. His weight was down to 96 pounds after his last operation, but has returned to 128 pounds. For most of his adult life Frank smoked 40 cigarettes a day; he has managed to cut down to 15. What bothers him as much as the pain is that his hands go dead—turning white and then blue—in cold weather.

Remarkably, Frank is still working, as an engine repairer for British Rail. "Isn't that heavy work?" the therapist asks. "No, they've put me on benchwork now. I can manage it, no problem." Clearly, Frank is attached to his work and it's an important factor in keeping up his morale. He takes morphine (MST) for the pain—"sometimes it works, sometimes it doesn't, I don't know why." The clinic has recommended electrical stimulation pads, but he doesn't find them effective, and in any case, they work loose when he's at the bench and interfere with his efficiency. He says that he would prefer to do without them, so Justins tells him that he has every right to make his own decisions and work out his own ways of coping with pain.

THE WHITTINGTON PAIN PROGRAM

At the Whittington, a general hospital in north London, some of the patients who have attended the pain clinic are invited to enroll in a 7-week program of pain management. There are eight people in each group, and all are people whose pain has defied every form of treatment that the hospital can offer; this program, they know, is the last resort.

Half an hour before the patients arrive, the professional team gathers for a discussion. Dr. John Skinner, a consultant anesthetist, is assisted by a clinical psychologist, a physician with special skill in hypnotism, an occupational therapist, and a physiotherapist.

This Wednesday, it's the sixth session of the seven. One patient has phoned to say that she's not coming; her explanation is that she's in too much pain. "I bet her husband has discouraged her," says the psychologist. "We can learn a lesson from that—we should have worked with him too." Nonattendance has been a problem with this group (it didn't occur with other groups). "They're an unusually intelligent lot," Skinner comments. "Maybe that's the trouble—they don't take anything on trust." Eventually, five of the eight show up.

Doris is an elderly woman wearing stylish tinted spectacles. Her speech is educated and precise, her clothes neat. She suffers from chronic neck pain.

Linda, a middle-aged woman, has neck pain too. She works behind the counter at the Social Security office. This is a bad period for her because her union has called a strike; normally, dealing with the problems of the claimants helps her not to think of the pain.

Jean, youngish and attractive, was born with a congenital hip deformity. "The others can remember being without pain," she remarks. "I've always been in pain. I don't know if that's an advantage or not."

Alice, a tall woman who gives an impression of physical strength, has worked all her adult life as a nurse and became a ward sister. She can give you the exact date, 2 years ago, when her problem started. As she was lifting a patient, she suddenly felt an agonizing pain in her back. She went home, expecting to take a week or two off work, but the pain has stayed with her ever since. She has been obliged to retire from work and spends her days at home, generally alone (her husband has a job and there are no children). For Alice, always an active and energetic person, the enforced idleness is a sore trial.

Bill's back pain came on more gradually, but is now very severe. He can hardly bear to sit on a chair and stands through most of the session, leaning on a stick; Bill and Alice both walk very slowly. Bill is a big, powerfully built man and one would guess that he has a background of manual work—perhaps he is a construction worker. Actually, he worked as a butler. It's now 7 years since he had to stop working.

The first session is with the doctor with skill in hypnotism. He induces a hypnotic state by instructing the patients to roll their eyes, as if trying to look at their own foreheads, and breathe deeply. Then he tells them: "Imagine you're in a very happy place. Imagine you're on the beach, sunbathing. Now imagine your left arm is attached to a balloon." Jean's arm rises two feet; she's in deep hypnosis. Linda's arm goes up a few inches. All the members of the group are hypnotized sufficiently to be open to suggestion. The doctor says: "You can do this for yourself. Every time you do it, you'll go deeper. My words will go into your mind. You'll feel stronger, more peaceful, calmer. You'll find it easier to do things. You'll have more control over your pain." Gradually, in silence, they emerge from the hypnotic state. Linda says, "That was fantastic."

Skinner and the occupational therapist join the group for a discussion on stress. Jean describes how angry she gets when someone jumps the line at the bank and when she sees people dropping litter. "I hate them all. I'd love to destroy them." Asked what she observes in herself on these occasions, she says: "My muscles tense, my voice is lower, I'm taking on a male attitude. It makes my pain worse."

Linda says that she's always calm and patient with the claimants (unlike her colleagues, she remarks), but she flares up with her husband and son. "I can't stand the boy cheeking me." Skinner tells her, "You clenched your fist as you said that."

Bill often uses the word "frustrated." "Silly little things like trying to wash the dishes—I can't do it, I get so frustrated." He goes into the bathroom to have a good swear. "Oh, we all swear," the others in the group assure him. There's some laughter about the words they use. Bill continues, "I get all upset for no apparent reason. It makes me very angry. My wife's threatened to leave me." This is said with an unconvincing laugh; it isn't clear whether it should be taken seriously.

The occupational therapist hands out a sheet headed *Perception of Stress*. It reads in part: "If you tell yourself you can't cope with a situation the likelihood is that you won't. Because you are thinking negatively it prevents you from thinking about solutions to the problem or ways that you could cope. . . . It is possible to retrain your thinking patterns and therefore your reaction to stresses."

The group splits up for individual talks with one of the staff members. The theme of this session is goal setting; last week, each patient chose a goal to be achieved. Skinner asks Jean, "Did you go swimming, then?" She admits that she didn't, because she was afraid of slipping at the pool. "Maybe you chose that goal because it was too ambitious," Skinner suggests. Her next goal will be to walk a given distance along the main road. She confides, "Finally I may be unable to walk at all. I can't bear to think of it." Skinner tells her, "I had a patient who was in a worse state than you, and he managed to run a mile."

Jean says, "There's such hopelessness in me, nothing works. I've run up against so many brick walls, I don't try any more." Her marriage is unhappy: "You know, I can do just about anything when my husband's away." She has tried to persuade her husband to visit a psychiatrist, but the suggestion threatens him and he refuses. "You could see a marriage guidance counselor yourself," Skinner says. Jean answers, "I just want to get rid of him, but I can't." However, Skinner says seriously that her next goal should be to see the counselor. Reluctantly, Jean agrees.

The next session is in the gym with the physiotherapist. The exercises are very demanding, but the therapist insists that everyone must keep trying. Doris does all the exercises successfully; a contented smile appears on her face. Alice is obviously in pain and says, "I can't do this, I just can't." The therapist says, "Do the best you can. Don't give up." No one is allowed to stand still or opt out.

The day ends with another discussion, this time led by the clinical psychologist. Pain control techniques are the subject— what does one do when a bad bout of pain is coming on? Jean says that she finds that deep, slow breathing helps more than anything else. Bill says that he has to lie down flat on the floor. "Are you sure you're not punishing yourself?" the psychologist asks, and he agrees that this is probably true. She suggests that it would be better to get into some activity that occupies the mind—painting, sketching, or simply reading an interesting book. "Reading doesn't accomplish anything," Bill objects. He sighs, "Still, you can't just watch the TV all day, can you?" Alice says that she's starting on a study project on homelessness together with some friends.

The program concludes with a discussion on whether it has been helpful. Doris: "Yes, I've got quite a different attitude now I've acquired some knowledge." Linda: "Oh, it's definitely helped. I came here as a last resort, and now I know that life isn't hopeless." Alice: "I was so much alone, Wednesday gave me something to look forward to. I'll always remember it." The best aspect, everyone agrees, was getting together with other people in pain. "It reminds you that you're not the only one in the world." Alice says. "People who don't have chronic pain just can't understand what it's like. They ask, 'How are you today?' and you have to answer, 'Oh, I'm fine.' So it's good to be with people who do understand."

Before separating, the participants in the program agree to keep in touch, talk regularly on the phone, and meet if possible. Those who are relatively mobile promise to visit the others. Even if nothing else has been achieved, they have made new friends, and that is sure to make life easier. Since the hospital keeps follow-up records on all the people who attend the pain clinic, it can be said a year later that the promises were kept and the friends were still in touch. The value of the program was inevitably limited—but definite and lasting.

THE HOSPICE IDEA (48, 55)

In most people's minds, severe pain is associated with very serious illness, leading to death. On the whole, this is an accurate perception. Pain does increase with damage to the body, especially to highly innervated structures. As we have seen, cancer is often painless in its early stages but is likely to cause pain as it advances. About 80% of people who die of cancer will suffer severe pain in the terminal stage, unless something is done to ward it off.

To die in pain is a terrible experience, which no one should be allowed to endure. Many a sufferer has longed for death, knowing the pain to be utterly pointless. If it is terrible for the patient, it is also very distressing for surviving relatives. Many a wife has cried out, "I know he must die, but why must he suffer like this?" Life in these conditions loses all dignity and meaning and ceases to be life in any true sense.

The idea of the hospice was generated to help people in this plight. In past centuries, the words "hospice" and "hospital" were almost synonymous. Both are defined in the *Oxford Dictionary* as "a place of rest"—for strangers and travelers, for the sick, for the old. It is only in modern times, with the development of intensive medicine aiming at cures, that the values of rest and care have been relegated to minor importance in hospitals.

It is appropriate for a patient to enter a hospice when death is extremely likely (doctors will never say that it is certain) and when active therapy aimed at cure or prolongation of life can no longer be recommended. This judgment can be made with considerable confidence in advanced cancer cases, but cannot be made in cases of heart disease, the other major cause of death. Consequently, most people admitted to hospices are cancer patients.

It should be stressed, however, that a hospice is not simply a place where people are made comfortable while they wait for death. It is the setting for medical practice of a highly skilled and sophisticated kind, currently in the process of steady improvement as knowledge advances. This branch of medicine is sometimes called palliative medicine, sometimes symptom control. Of the symptoms to be brought under control, the most important is obviously pain, but others include nausea and vomiting, anorexia, constipation, incontinence, and coughing. Medical techniques exist to control all these conditions.

The first institution to use the term "hospice" with application to the care of the dying was founded in Lyon, France, in 1842. Others gradually came into existence; St. Joseph's Hospice in the East End of London was founded by the Irish Sisters of Charity in 1905. Dr. (now Dame) Cicely Saunders worked there for a number of years, introducing new methods of pain control. She began to make plans for a hospice that would be housed in a well-equipped modern building, would be a base for home care as well as the care of inpatients, and would also be a center for research and teaching. As a result of an energetic fund-raising effort, St. Christopher's Hospice in south London was built and was opened in 1967. Dame Cicely was its medical director until her recent retirement.

The philosophy of St. Christopher's, in Dame Cicely's words, is: "Terminal suffering should be approached as an illness in itself, one that will respond to rationally based treatment" (55). Fear and anxiety are seen as central problems; she notes that "if fear is aroused it will immediately enhance pain by tension." Symptom control, she explains, "does not mean an implicit "there is nothing more that we can do," but an explicit "everything possible is being done." The promise to the patient is: "We will do all we can not only to help you to die peacefully, but also to live until you die."

The question of frankness is one that has been much debated by doctors and other hospice workers. The human capacity for denial is stronger than one might perhaps expect. In a recent survey of patients entering St. Christopher's, 30% knew that they were dying, 45% knew that they had cancer but had no definite expectation concerning the outcome, and 25%

were quite unaware of what the trouble was. Once in the hospice, the patient will naturally observe that others in nearby beds have died. (Hospices generally provide four-bed rooms, though single rooms are available when preferred.) The best policy, it has been found, is to wait until the patient puts a question and then to say: "Yes, we think you will soon die." A study has been made comparing institutions employing this policy of frankness with others choosing a policy of reticence. It was found that the former had "less anxious and depressed patients."

Since the terminal stage of cancer is clearly recognizable, the policy of frankness risks few surprises. Some patients do, however, show remarkable tenacity, especially when pain is brought under control. Records of patients at St. Christopher's show 5% surviving for 6 months or more, the longest period being 6 years.

American experience has been similar (50). The first American hospice, founded in 1974, was Hospice of Connecticut, which had a home care team. Thousands of patients are now cared for along these lines—some in independent institutions such as Hospice of Connecticut, the majority in specialized wards or departments within hospitals. American terminology draws a distinction between "closed awareness" (knowledge of the terminal condition is withheld from the patient), "suspicion awareness" (the patient fishes for information to confirm suspicions of the terminal condition, and this is given in reply to questions) and "open awareness" (patients, family members, and hospice staff all know the full facts). There is general agreement that open awareness is the best policy. It cannot free the patient entirely from fear—not to fear death is hard indeed—but it alleviates the anxiety that derives from ignorance and bewilderment.

Most people with terminal cancer would choose to spend their last days at home, rather than in a hospital or even a hospice. Hence, an important part of the work of the hospice is to train nurses (based either at the hospice or at a hospital) who can effect symptom control for patients at home, and also to instruct family members in the relevant techniques. There is, of course, some flexibility about what is feasible; a patient may spend Monday to Friday in the hospice and go home for the weekend. Of patients entering St. Christopher's 20% are discharged. This means, in most cases, that they die at home within a short time.

An American writer actively involved in the hospice movement has observed the experiences and interpreted the feelings of the terminally ill. Among these was Ruth, described as "a tiny woman who appeared to be in her sixties and looked like a survivor of a concentration camp . . . painfully thin, with sunken cheeks and hollow eyes." The writer quotes a conversation between Ruth and a social worker in the hospice:

> Ruth: "I'm so bored, I need something to do."
> Social worker: "How about reading? Would you like a book?"
> Ruth: "No, it's hard to hold a book, they're so heavy."
> Social worker: "I can get you talking books and a machine to play them on."
> Ruth: "Oh, thank you, that would be great."

A remarkable account of hospice methods is given in *A Way to Die*, by Rosemary and Victor Zorza, whose daughter Jane died of cancer in 1976 at the age of 26 (77). She suffered severe pain in the hospital, and a doctor is quoted as telling her father: "There's nothing we could do about her pain. It's something she must expect in a case like this." Later, we read:

> Jane had now been moved into the farthest corner of the ward where the nurses seldom passed. They would come to administer the painkillers, but only after all the other patients had been taken care of, even if Jane had been ready and crying for a pill long before. They had strict orders that the pills were to be given every two or three hours, so, to be on the safe side, they made it every three.

Jane was brought home from the hospital and then, thanks to an understanding general practitioner, admitted to a hospice. She arrived in agonizing pain and mental anguish so severe that the hospice staff had never seen anything like it before. She was at once given so much heroin that a visiting doctor expected it to kill her, but in fact it conquered the pain. Thereafter, she was given injections in time to forestall the pain, and this freed her from the fear of experiencing pain before relief. As the hospice doctor explained: "You don't wait until the pain returns. You want to prevent this, to get on top and keep ahead of pain. . . . The idea is that you give the next dose before the effect of the previous one has worn off." This treatment raised Jane's morale and reduced the intensity of the pain so effectively that milder doses could be given. She said farewell to her family and friends in a composed manner and went to a tranquil death. Her parents write: "For us the memory is not one of pain and anguish but of her calm smile and peace of mind." However, it is terrible to think of the pain that Jane might have undergone in the 8 days that elapsed between her hospital experience and her death.

Two other true stories from hospice life are worth telling. At Edenhall Hospice in north London, an improbable but close friendship was formed between two men in terminal cancer. One was an unskilled laborer, the other an antique dealer who had written poetry throughout his life. The idea of writing poems had never occurred to the laborer, but in the closing phase of his life he wrote a score of them; one was evoked by his friend's death. He himself died soon afterward, but he had ended his life on an unexpected note of achievement.

A young woman of 28 had been married for about 10 months when she entered St. Christopher's. She had probably been suffering from cancer on her wedding day, but there was a fatal delay in the diagnosis, due partly to her own hesitation in seeing a doctor and partly to medical bungling. When she was admitted to hospital, the cancer was inoperable and incurable. She lay curled up in bed, unable to make the effort to move or speak. After transferring to St. Christopher's, she started getting out of bed and walking short distances and declared that she felt much better, although she was visibly nearer to death. Her husband, the staff, and other patients gathered for a party on the first wedding anniversary, an occasion of genuine happiness.

The level of care, constant attention, and effective pain control achieved in a hospice would obviously be impossible without a high staffing ratio. St. Christopher's, with 62 beds, has seven doctors, 90 nurses, and a total payroll of 230. There are also 350 unpaid volunteers who give varying amounts of time; this system is a valuable link with the surrounding community. Physiotherapy and occupational therapy are provided. At Edenhall, the range of activities includes gardening, painting and drawing, fabric printing, and clay modeling. Many patients have written or dictated their memories, leaving behind useful material for social historians.

Despite the high staffing ratio, hospices are money-savers. It has been shown that the cost of a hospice bed is between 50% and 70% of the cost of a hospital bed. This results from the absence of high-tech medicine, and of tests and treatments that are no longer appropriate.

The costs of running a hospice are mainly supplied by charitable foundations or raised in the community by the hospice itself. The National Health Service makes a contribution, varying in different parts of Britain but averaging 27%. There are 15 hospices wholly funded by the National Health Service (NHS). Patients are normally referred from an NHS hospital or by a general practitioner; they are never asked to pay anything.

Since St. Christopher's opened its doors, other hospices have been started all over Britain. But, in Dame Cicely Saunders' view, there is no point in aiming to build a hospice in every small town. It is far more desirable to spread the hospice idea—to get the philosophy and the methods of palliative medicine accepted by hospitals and doctors. There are now 124 hospices in the strict sense of buildings bearing that name, but this does not count hospital departments working on hospice principles or hospice-trained home care teams.

In the United States, the hospice idea has been spreading since the 1970s (50). In the early days, it was handicapped by stringent rules adopted by Medicare and Medicaid, and also by Blue Cross and Blue Shield. Conservative medical opinion distrusted hospices as an unorthodox variant on regular hospital methods, while legislators feared that hospices, with their generous staffing and their more liberal use of drugs, would be intolerably expensive. These fears were dispelled by a 6-month study made by Methodist Hospital in Jacksonville, Florida, which set up a hospice program for some of its gravely ill patients, all dependent on Medicare. It was found that the average patient treated under the traditional system was spending 26 days in hospital at a daily cost of $309, but a patient in a hospice had an average stay of 11 days at a daily cost of $162. The hospice patients were able to spend more time at home, at an average daily cost to Medicare of only $16.40 plus $35 for each visit from a trained nurse. These figures were convincing, and in 1981 Congress passed legislation making hospice treatment available under Medicare. This was important, because 70% of hospice patients require Medicare support, while only 30% can pay from private insurance or out of their pockets.

Today, there are about a thousand hospice programs in the United States, including hospices in the full sense, hospital departments, and home care agencies. They are found in almost every state.

Around the world, there are hospices in 36 other nations from Argentina to Norway and from Jamaica to Japan. Sadly, but not surprisingly, they are found almost exclusively in the wealthy parts of the world. India, with its vast population, has only one hospice, and Indonesia has one. Throughout the Third World, terminal cancer patients suffering severe pain are spending their last days in inadequately equipped hospitals, or more often in their homes without any kind of professional care or pain-reducing drugs.

Pain clinics and hospices have a significance that extends beyond the strictly practical. They demonstrate the unity of mind and body, the inextricable relationship between anxiety and pain, and the contribution that can be made by various health professionals on an interdisciplinary basis—the sum being always more than the parts. They teach the lesson that there is never just nothing to be done about pain. They presage, we hope and trust, a better future.

12

Lessons and Prospects

We have surveyed the present situation with regard to pain, its victims, and those who fight it. Now we can turn to the future and ask what is likely to happen, and what tactics and strategy might be adopted by individuals and by groups.

BREAKING THE SILENCE

Already it seems extraordinary that the misery of vast numbers of people should be blanketed by a social silence. The hopeful aspect is that the very reasons for that silence contain its cure. We are witnessing a growing revolt by patients, by their friends and families, and by therapists. A sign of this revolt is the migration of patients away from orthodox medicine to explore the resources of ancient folk remedies. There is a basic rationality in the orthodox procedure of ignoring symptoms to concentrate on fundamental cure. But, while methods of cure are being discovered, everything that modern knowledge has to offer should be mobilized to deal with the symptoms too. Old ideas are changing in three ways that relate to the problem of pain.

First, we now challenge the acceptance of the miseries of life—death and taxes, disease and famine—as inevitable afflictions that must be borne with fortitude. Sophisticated thinkers, such as St. Augustine and, in our time, C. S. Lewis, have tried to represent this sad acceptance as a valuable property of human nature. They saw pain as the necessary price of a life that allowed the freedom of creativity. But, since the beginning of the twentieth century, all sorts of individuals and political groups—liberals, socialists, scientists, and campaigners—have refused to accept the dictates of inevitability. Their efforts have actually achieved, in some countries at least, drastically reduced death rates and sufficient food and shelter for the whole population, so that minds can be turned to consider the quality of life rather than mere survival. Those who have reached this stage (still a luxury for most of the world) can set their sights on positive health instead of an avoidance of disease, and comfort instead of an avoidance of misery. The emphasis now is on an improved environment, and on the concerns voiced by the green or ecological movement. It can be argued that such ambitions are premature while we have yet, on a global scale, to conquer the ancient scourges: war, famine, and pestilence. But the new outlook is certainly positive, and it fits perfectly with a refusal to accept the inevitability of pain.

A second change in contemporary thinking concerns the status of authority. The two centuries that have passed since the American and French revolutions can be regarded as an era of growing confidence in the ability of ordinary people to question the beneficence of authority. The basis of all traditional authority is enshrined in dogma, but the philosophy of the Age of Reason, coupled with the scientific method, provided the equipment to examine the validity of the dogma. The pontiffs and pundits (in every sphere, including the medical) are still on duty, seeking to preserve dogma by detecting heretical thoughts, but through these two centuries their power has been steadily weakened. A good example was the classical dogma that pain was beneficial and protective, as well as irrelevant to the aims and functions of medicine. Scientists and clinicians have produced strong evidence to set against these articles of faith.

Since pain was excluded from thorough investigation, the classical mechanism of a direct alarm system from tissue to brain was believed to explain everything. This dogmatic model has been rejected in favor of a more subtle understanding, which integrates mind and body and incorporates pain in a dynamic system of behavior.

Through most of human history, the individual faced with a problem—such as the appearance of pain—turned to authority for a solution, or at least for consolation. In return, authority demanded respect, implicit trust, and obedience. Authority over pain was shared between priests and doctors (sometimes the same men). This unquestioned dominance of authority belongs, or should belong, to the past. But old habits die hard, and authority is seldom willingly surrendered.

The third change is in the sphere of responsibility. A study was made of what doctors said to amputees suffering from chronic pain (56, 57). Two percent of military amputees and 47% of civilian amputees were told that nothing could be done for them. The most charitable interpretation of this flat statement is that the doctor had no specific cure to offer from the resources of his particular specialty. A more critical interpretation is that the patient was simply being dismissed and told that his duty was to endure the pain. This is no longer acceptable. The responsibility of the doctor, stated as a minimum, is to mobilize every possible resource to cope with the problem. The patient need no longer be left in isolation, with technical ignorance as an excuse. Amputees have banded together in self-help groups, partly to supply companionship and understanding, but also to put pressure on doctors, scientists, charities, and governments, and thus to ensure that they are not forgotten. Tolstoy's peg-legged victims of the Crimea lived in a society that counseled resignation to suffering, and political activism was certainly not a custom among old soldiers. At best, they may have been the recipients of paternalistic charity. A different attitude prevails among the amputees of Vietnam—and, let us hope, the amputees of Afghanistan.

The study we have cited also found that 5% of the veterans and 9% of the civilians were told that the pain would go away of its own accord. This does occasionally happen, but the statement would be met with derision by a World War II amputee who has been in pain for 45 years. Twenty-four percent of the amputees perceived that doctors avoided an answer to their questions. Worst of all, the majority in both groups were told that the pain was imaginary. This cruelest of statements transfers the responsibility for pain from the patient's body, which the doctor regards as his proper concern, to the patient's mind, which is (in the view of this kind of doctor) none of his business. It also neatly, and authoritatively, transfers blame and responsibility from doctor to patient. It is a perfect recipe for generating feelings of guilt, helplessness, and isolation. Not only does the doctor decline to hear any more nonsensical complaints, but the patient is warned to keep his hallucinations to himself and not to inflict them on friends and relatives.

Often, the guilt and anger thus induced lead the patient to ask: "Why me?" The atavistic interpretation of pain as punishment lies deep within us all. An introspective spiral of self-doubt completes the patient's isolation in a prison of his own making—but constructed, in the first place, by society. Smashing that Bastille is the aim of the revolution in attitude and therapy now in progress.

The prospect is by no means grim. A breath of fresh air is blowing across the rubbish dump of inhumanity. The best example is surely the hospice movement, which has outlawed the phrase: "There is nothing more to be done." The hospice outlook goes well beyond the customary concept of tender loving care. The word "care," one of the most beautiful in the language, is nowadays one of the most devalued and is used to mean "We recognize the existence of a problem and propose to do absolutely nothing about it." Hospices aim not only to care, but to bring together every resource from love to scientific skill for the benefit of their patients. Similarly, pain clinics aim to relieve patients of the responsibility of shopping around from specialist to specialist and present them with an integrated treatment program combining everything that is available for the relief of pain.

Even governments are changing their attitudes. The United States, through the National Institutes of Health (NIH) and the National Science Foundation, is responsible for probably almost half of the fundamental biomedical research in the world. The NIH remains subdivided into institutes dedicated to the cure of the traditional disease targets, such as cancer, heart disease, and arthritis. They are justified by their past and present success. But, within many of these subdivisions classified according to disease, there are growing programs of symptom management, especially pain projects. There is also an increasing recognition of the role of neglected professionals, such as nurses, who cope with real day-to-day problems while physicians, surgeons, and scientists indulge in dreams of high-tech fundamental solutions.

Other countries often trail behind the United States in the percentage of national wealth devoted to medical problems. Each has its central source of research funds, but in general, they are more traditional in the pursuit of ultimate solutions. One might have hoped that poorer countries would be more pragmatic and would look for today's answers to today's problems. Unfortunately, they are all too often dedicated to grossly ambitious fundamental projects, far beyond their intellectual or financial resources. Ordinary citizens, especially those in pain, could assume a constructive role by demanding a more realistic use of governmental funds—for instance, the testing and validation of folk remedies.

Next to governments, private charities have had a crucial role in funding and guiding medical research and educational efforts. As with official programs, they concentrate on the search for cures of diseases—the obvious ones are again cancer, heart disease, and arthritis—but may also get involved in something like the Riley–Day syndrome which most people have never heard of. The charities too are beginning to admit the need for symptomatic treatment as well as cure. For example, the International Spinal Research Trust is dedicated to finding a cure for paraplegia. This worthy aim will require a solution to the problem of why axons in the central nervous system do not regenerate, which demands a deep understanding of the biology of nerve cells. Thus, the charity is encouraging and funding some very subtle and laborious basic studies. Meanwhile, it recognizes that paraplegics are often in pain, and that it may be easier to solve the pain problems than to achieve the ultimate aim of restoring sensation and movement.

However, among the many admirable specialized charities working on an international scale, only one is dedicated primarily to the problem of pain and to research and education in the field of pain. This is the International Pain Foundation.

In the medical world, it is clear that there is a new wave of interest in the subject of pain. We have mentioned the International Association for the Study of Pain, whose members include about 4000 scientists and clinicians from all over the world. It publishes a monthly research journal, and there are about 10 other journals for particular interest groups or in different languages. The first textbooks are appearing. Always a matter of human and social need, pain has become a subject of academic importance.

The pharmaceutical companies, obviously, have a special role and responsibility. In 1988, Bristol Myers initiated a handsome annual prize for achievement in pain research and chose one of the authors (P.D.W.) as the first recipient. This company is also making 5-year grants, amounting to $250,000 each, to the five most distinguished research teams in the United States.

WHERE ARE THE SCIENTISTS GOING?

We see, therefore, that pain research is on the move. Now we must inquire into the direction of the movement—an important question not only for professionals, but also for people in pain.

Scientists are a surprisingly conservative bunch. It is their custom to explore a classical theory to the limit before abandoning it in favor of a new line of thought. The classical theory of neural mechanisms was seductive and simple. It assumed that nerve cells were dedicated to special functions, one of these being pain. It was implicit that the nerve cells established stable connections. Let us pause here to discuss this concept of stability.

There is no doubt that, in general, the functioning of the brain is remarkably stable. To say that it is normal, under a wide range of circumstances, to feel a given stimulus as painful is to make a statement of stability. But there are two ways to achieve stability. One is to construct a rigid structure of piling one brick on another and connecting them with mortar, or whatever may be suitable in the context. The other way is through the continuous dynamic interaction of opposing forces. This is how an airplane maintains a stable altitude and course, while flying on an autopilot. Scientists today are reluctantly revising their understanding of the stability of pain-producing mechanisms.

The autopilot requires the existence of hard-wired, reliable inputs that report on factors such as engine speed. It is connected to rigid outputs that adjust, for instance, the rudder angle. The brain, similarly, needs reliable rigid inputs and outputs. The question for the scientist is how the input is linked to the output. In the classical theory of pain, the rigidity of the input was continued by rigid links to the output. Now, we are unraveling a complex of dynamic interacting links. Thus it was that we arrived at the concept of gate control.

To dissect such a complex is naturally far more difficult than to locate a continuous thread or wire. Its dynamic properties make it elusive, because the state of the components changes while they are being examined. The problems are multiplied as it becomes apparent that, as well as the gate controls, which are operating in milliseconds, there are at least two other, slower controls. Changes in the pain system associated with spreading tenderness take minutes to appear and last for hours. Later changes mediated by chemical transport controls operate on a time scale of days or months. To arrive at a full analysis of all these controls will demand not only a great deal of hard work, but also subtlety, cleverness, and inventiveness.

Of the new sciences, molecular biology is making the most rapid advances. It is capable of analyzing and synthesizing the finest details of the components of living systems. This immensely powerful new field has only one weakness. Its scientists are inevitably dependent on an understanding of the systems they propose to dissect. They were very happy as long as they were told by classical theory that there were nerves labeled as pain nerves. That was something to get their teeth into. But if pain occurs as a result of dynamic interactions, then the finest analysis of a single component will tell us no more about the pain process than the analysis of the strings of a Stradivarius will tell us about a violin concerto. It would be interesting, useful, and even commercially profitable, but it would make only a minor contribution.

The obvious allies of the molecular biologists are the pharmacologists and the pharmaceutical industry, who are literally in the business of molecules. They are also in the business of making money, as they are reminded by accountants whose duty is to ensure a return on investment. To launch a new drug is an enormously costly and prolonged process of trials, tests, licenses, manufacture, and advertising. Early in this century, the drug companies were genuine innovators. In the last 50 years, they have produced no real innovation in the field of pain relief, notwithstanding the firework display of advertising hype that greets every minor variant on an existing drug. The problem is that to hope for a practicable and profitable outcome from a piece of basic research is a wild gamble, and the use of company funds for long-odds bets is inhibited, if not prohibited.

In this situation, the responsibility for genuine innovation falls on the universities. They too, however, are under financial pressure to win battles in the marketplace. Meanwhile, people in pain are waiting. They rightly demand that society should find the resources in one way or another.

The struggle against pain is not the equivalent of putting a man on the moon. That was done by collecting and applying the existing knowledge. To learn to help people in pain, we need new knowledge which does not yet exist, and which could be combined with what we already possess. This does not mean that research money should be scattered at random to bright applicants with a good line of talk. It does mean that we should encourage investigators to stop dotting the i's and crossing the t's of the last decade's research, and to seek a new dimension of understanding of the nervous system and its pain-producing mechanisms.

Another and very different group of thinkers has its own role to play. These are the psychologists, linguists, and philosophers. Now that we know that pain is not a simple consequence of sticking in a pin, we must deal with the fact that the pain has an impact on an individual with a past, a present, and a future. The intrusion of the pin (or the tooth extraction or the amputation) can be defined as an event without reference to the person concerned, but this person will be different every time. Some of us are inclined to fight when in trouble, and others to flight. Some are always investigating and analyzing the outer world, while others turn to inner contemplation. There are creative dreamers, and there are practical achievers. It is not conceivable that all these people would react identically to a given event.

To take an example—but it is a large example with almost infinite depth—each person varies from each other person in the use of language. As a method of communication, language depends on the characteristics of the speaker and the listener, and on what the speaker thinks that the listener wishes (or deserves) to hear. Linguists can tell us much, and in the future should be able to tell us more, about the uses and functions of language as a form of behavior. And the more we know about the behavior of people in pain, the more we shall understand about pain.

All this will need a great deal of hard work and clear thinking. At present, some schools of psychology are producing quantities of mindless verbiage unlikely to generate useful ideas. We shall achieve nothing by classifying people in fixed categories to which we extend approval or disapproval. Studies of behavior, however, do have a constructive therapeutic aspect, which can be developed, and which goes beyond the identification of "people at risk."

Some people have an exceptional ability to escape from hard, objective reality into an imaginative sphere. They are swept away by music into another world. They emerge from the theater or the movies with a changed gait and expression, still identifying with a character who attracts or impresses them. These innocent quirks are strongly associated with a placebo reaction. Could we find ways to help prosaic, uptight people to enjoy their dreams? It could be very beneficial for people in pain.

There are some people whose attention mechanisms are orderly, stable, and rigid. There are others who flit easily from one focus of attention to another. The latter, when in pain, react well to distraction therapies and strategies of coping. Can we teach people to switch attention more rapidly, without turning them into silly, vapid butterflies? These are some of the opportunities that await behavioral scientists, but they will depend on a much deeper understanding of such attributes as attention, speech, mood, and meaning.

PHYSICIAN, HEAL THYSELF

Doctors have the reputation of being pompous and insensitive (as well as greedy). They are in serious need of reexamining their public reputation. Yet they are the guardians of an enormous storehouse of knowledge and skill; we cannot do without them.

The successes of the medical profession in diagnosis and therapy have generated a demand for curative medicine which no society can meet. Doctors, therefore, are seen as the controllers of a rationing system that decrees that some are served and others neglected. The consumers, as they have become more informed and sophisticated, have also grown more suspicious; a neurosurgeon in Miami pays an annual $250,000 insurance premium before he can pick up a scalpel. Insurance companies and governments, who are the main sources of medical funds, apply a cost–benefit analysis to ensure that diagnosis and treatment are worth the investment. What hope is there for the patient who has no diagnosis on the approved list of diseases and no prospect of cure, but is simply in pain?

This self-generated destruction by success has led to a manifest deterioration of the medical profession. A recent American survey investigated the job satisfaction of middle-aged doctors. Most of them had long ago lost their pride in service to suffering humanity and were harried by the increasing demands and suspicions of patients accusing them of incompetence and chicanery. It is no wonder that the numbers of applicants to medical schools are falling.

In the nineteenth century, the leading physicians and surgeons were not only respected pillars of society, but also innovative thinkers whose ideas we still find stimulating. To cite only British doctors who had enlightening ideas about pain, Sir David Ferrier, Sir Frederick Mott, Sir Henry Head, and Sir Thomas Lewis were scientific giants, and their knighthoods show that they were appreciated by the political and social establishment of their time. These men had time to think, and to work at research as well as at their clinical duties. Today, no one could put forward a name to match this list, despite the vast increase both in the stock of knowledge and in the numbers of the profession.

No recent Nobel Prize laureates in medicine have been clinicians, and very few have had even basic medical degrees. The torch has passed to the scientists. This was already evident in the 1940s when Johns Hopkins, one of the most famous medical schools, appointed a researcher, Philip Bard, Ph.D., as Dean. As a consequence, the ambition of the medical graduate is to achieve rapid success as a carpenter or plumber on a high technological (and high income) level. The style that characterizes these graduates reflects their class origins and the intensity of the technological brainwashing to which they have been subjected. Walking in their white coats, with the stethoscope carefully in evidence, they are able to view patients as inferior beings. Their attitudes merely reflect the values imbibed from their seniors.

Somehow, clinicians must be rescued from the trap into which they have been led. They desperately need time in which to consider individual patients and human problems. Let us take the growing problem of postherpetic neuralgia, for which there is at present no treatment. It is a growing problem because it is most common in old people, whose numbers (thanks partly to the successes of medicine) are steadily increasing. This extremely painful and crippling condition begins as an acute attack of shingles (herpes zoster). A painful burning rash appears, generally on one side of the face or chest. In most cases, it dies down and disappears in a week or so, but a minority of patients experience a chronic burning pain with exquisite tenderness, which lasts for the rest of their lives. Most doctors, knowing that the condition is likely to disappear, prescribe aspirin and a cooling ointment and cross their fingers. Some attack it more vigorously with antiviral agents and with nerve blocks, which completely stop the acute pain. There are strong indications that this treatment prevents the progress of the acute condition into the chronic state. Such indications have been known for 40 years, but no clinicians have investigated whether this is a definite fact.

Why not? The treatment is expensive and skilled. To evaluate its success would take time, money, and effort, which have not been made available. It would be necessary to collect large numbers of patients from widely scattered physicians, admit them to hospitals for an agreed treatment procedure, and follow them for years. This is perfectly feasible, but it is obviously expensive and it involves educating the doctors who encounter the patients in the first place. Suppose, however, that this action is taken and proves that the treatment prevents the chronic pain. Should we then be ready and able to give the treatment to all cases of shingles in order to assist the minority who develop postherpetic neuralgia? That problem is not medical but social.

We could cite many similar problems that cannot be solved only by physicians and surgeons. The social responsibility is to liberate doctors so that they can do what they know they should do—and then discover new problems and work out new solutions.

A THERAPEUTIC COMMUNITY

We have been assuming that every person in pain has consulted a qualified doctor. In reality, this is far from being the case; our society includes subcultures of totally disenchanted people who are opposed to mainstream science and medicine. Their outlook can be understood, but they may be the sufferers if they reject the abilities of orthodox doctors. Doctors can (and, when in good form, do) make precise, unequivocal diagnoses and prognoses. They can prescribe treatment, and we have seen that some kinds of pain respond very satisfactorily to orthodox treatments, while others are reduced to a tolerable level. Finally, doctors can give clear advice on the type of activity that is safe. This is important for the patient who wishes to set reasonable targets, for the physiotherapist, and indeed for the peace of mind and safety of the "alternative" therapist.

Patients who consult doctors too often, however, are as ill advised as those who never do so. Pain is by its nature obsessive, but it is worse when combined with the obsessive conviction that someone, somewhere, must have the answer. Surgeons are a particular target for the demand that the pain can, literally, be cut out. An angry, aggressive patient can mobilize enormous psychological pressure on therapists to "do something." The endless search can be as sad and dangerous as that of a medieval pilgrim tramping the roads in quest of salvation.

One might expect patients to learn about what is feasible and beneficial. Some do learn. It is a pleasure to see a patient who has responded well to a hip replacement returning with a logical request for an operation on the other hip when it becomes arthritic. That is in contrast with the patient who has had 10 back operations and has found yet another doctor to whom he presents a thick file of notes, reports, and X-rays. The specialist, thus challenged, is tempted to join the patient and agree that the 10 previous surgeons didn't know their business. On the other hand, to refuse the request is to add to the anger and isolation of the obsessed patient, and perhaps to leave him to the tender mercies of quacks and confidence tricksters.

The extremes of pain behavior present a very sad picture. There is, however, a common problem which affects everyone who is in pain for long periods. This problem concerns the meaning of the word "acceptance." It is one thing to accept that no one has a complete solution to this particular pain condition. It is quite another thing to accept that nothing can be done. To demand that the patient should accept the uselessness of all help is to condemn him to a feeling of betrayal, alienation, and depression. The result is a downward spiral, which becomes increasingly difficult to interrupt. The hospice movement teaches us a splendid example by asserting and proving that comfort and dignity can be achieved even for those whose life is ending.

Let us remind the reader here of the Chinese doctrine of recruiting the patient as a member of his own treatment team, so that patients and therapists become comrades in the best sense of the word, with its connotations of shared respect and responsibility. In Western hospitals, dominated by accountants' demands for cost-effectiveness and efficiency, a patient is lucky to be given a bed the night before an operation; he is more likely to be ordered to present himself, breakfastless, on the morning of the crucial day. The reassuring old concept of the bedside manner has disappeared, since the patient is aware of no one near the bed but a swirl of anonymous, often masked figures. Patients say, indeed, that they have had fuller and more helpful conversations with the ambulance crew or the ward cleaner than with doctors and nurses. Contemporary pressures have distanced the patient from the therapist and produced an exaggerated belief in instant solutions. Perhaps we need to train our professionals in the specialty of cooperation with the patient.

What is needed, in particular, is the creation of a therapeutic community centered on the individual patient. People who are not officially classified as highly trained are certainly capable of assuming more responsibility than they are now given. Nurses, district nurses and health visitors, physiotherapists and occupational therapists, and ancillaries of various kinds have too often been arbitrarily restricted and denied the chance to use their full potential. Patient groups, formed to complain of medical neglect, have developed as mutual self-help teams. The complexities of sophisticated medicine mean that, even in the most affluent of societies, we cannot leave it to the specialist to do all that is needful. We must take on do-it-yourself responsibilities, which require education, acceptance, and encouragement.

To issue a command to "pull yourself together" to a deeply depressed, inactive patient is an obscenity. The condition of such patients is predictable and preventable, since they were plunged into it by a sequence of dismissal and neglect. They can be rescued only by great imaginative effort as well as professional help. Sometimes, the outcome of neglect is suicide.

A suicide by a person who is unnecessarily depressed is, clearly, a tragic event and should evoke guilt in those who had stood by. We feel differently, no doubt, when a person with a perfectly clear mind, beyond recovery from a terminal illness, decides that his useful life has come to an end and that his future lacks purpose or dignity. It is a crime to assist a suicide, but there is little doubt that it is covertly practiced while authority looks the other way. Moral problems about what is right, what is wrong, and what is pardonable are never simple.

CONCLUSION

We have written this book as a contribution to a greater understanding of pain, because the experiences of a person in pain depend significantly on his beliefs about it. Some common beliefs are unconstructive and harmful—that pain inevitably grows worse; that it is a mystery beyond comprehension; that no one, including the sufferer, can do anything about it; or that it is his own fault. These beliefs are not only false; they constitute self-fulfilling prophecies and contribute to a bad outlook. They must be challenged and indeed attacked. Obviously it is best when people question their own beliefs, but sometimes they need encouragement.

Only when victims of pain work themselves free from these beliefs—above all, the belief that nothing can be done—can they take steps toward liberation from pain. The first step is regaining the possibility of physical activity. It may well be, literally, the first step: that is, getting out of bed and putting a foot on the floor. Against all expectation, movement itself reduces pain. It reverses the physiological decline that results from inactivity. It generates a sense of well-being. It is a distraction from passive concentration on pain.

The next goal is to reawaken a sense of expectation—an orientation toward the future. Expectation may take the shape of fantasy and fancy, of dreams that cannot yet be realized, but this is all to the good. Children build happiness from their fantasies of invisible friends, talking animals, and frogs that turn into princes. We adults are much too adult; we need to relearn how to daydream, how to surrender ourselves to thoughts and feelings that do not derive from cautious calculation. When the mind is riveted to pain, this can be hard work. But it opens the door to placebo responses—in other words, to responding with hope and confidence to every kind of assistance.

The third goal is exploration. It is difficult to pursue because it is the opposite of the inactivity inherent in depression. Among other effects, depression influences the attitude to medicines. Failure to take medicines as prescribed, and failure to do the exercises prescribed by the physiotherapist, are very common among people in pain. The lack of compliance may be caused by a rejection of authority, but in most cases it is derived from a conviction that nothing will do any good. When the person who has achieved a positive attitude toward exploration takes medicine (or exercise, or food), he does so not to obey orders, but because he is actively exploring their possibilities.

Expectation, exploration, and the discarding of hampering beliefs are all feasible, but are much more likely to be attained when the patient has some support. Isolation is the worst of handicaps; a therapeutic community is a reality even when it is a community of two. But the process is reciprocal, for a positive outlook on the part of the patient invites and encourages support.

What matters, above all, is that we should look to the future. We shall never abolish pain; the human body is so constructed that a sprained ankle or a blow on the head is bound to hurt. What we can overcome is a hopeless, helpless imprisonment within immutable pain. In the 1990s, we know that we have a much greater power to do this than at any earlier time in history. We must resolve, year by year and incessantly, to advance humanity's power over pain.

References

1. AITKEN-SWAN, J. (1959) The frequency of pain in terminal cancer. *Practitioner*, 183: 64–72.
2. ANNAN, G. (1988) Roughing it. *N. Rev. Books*, 35: 3–4.
3. ATKINSON, J. H., *et al.* (1988) Depressed mood in chronic low back pain. *Pain*, 35: 47–60.
4. BACH, S., NORENG, M. F., & TJELLDEN, N. U. (1988) Phantom limb pains in amputees. *Pain*, 33: 297–301.
5. BAXTER, D. W., & OLSZEWSKI, J. (1960) Congenital insensitivity to pain. *Brain*, 83: 381–393.
6. BEECHER, H. K. (1959) *The Measurement of Subjective Responses.* Oxford University Press, New York.
7. BONICA, J. J. (1953) *The Management of Pain.* Lea & Febiger, Philadelphia.
8. BONICA, J. J., & CHADWICK, H. S. (1989) Labour pain. In: *The Textbook of Pain*, 2nd ed., P. D. Wall & R. Melzack, eds. Churchill Livingstone, Edinburgh.
9. BORING, E. G. (1963) *The Physical Dimensions of Consciousness.* Dover, New York.
10. BROMAGE, P. R., & MELZACK, R. (1974) Phantom limbs and the body schema. *Canad. Anaesth. Soc. J.*, 21: 267–274.
11. BRUYN, G. W. (1983) Epidemiology of migraine. *Headache*, 23: 127–133.
12. CAMPBELL, S. (1988) Silent myocardial ischaemia. *Brt. Med. J.*, 297: 751–752.
13. CARLEN, P., WALL, P. D., NADVORNA, H., & STEINBACH, T. (1978) Phantom limbs and related phenomena in recent traumatic amputations. *Neurology*, 28: 211–217.
14. CHOINIERE, M. (1989) The pain of burns. In: *The Textbook of Pain*, P. D. Wall & R. Melzack, eds. Churchill Livingstone, Edinburgh.

15. CORNWALL, A., & DANDERI, D. C. (1988) The effect of experimentally induced anxiety on the experience of pressure pain. *Pain*, 35: 105–115.
16. DESCARTES, R. (1644) *L'Homme*. Paris.
17. DICK READ, G. (1944) *Childbirth without Fear*. Harper, New York.
18. ECCLES, J. C. (1980) *The Human Psyche*. Springer, Berlin.
19. EURIPEDES. "Medea," lines 248–251.
20. FINNESON, B. E. (1969) *Diagnosis and Management of Pain Syndromes*. Saunders, Philadelphia.
21. FLANNERY, R., *et al.* (1981) Ethnicity as a factor in the expression of pain. *Psychosomatics*, 22: 39–50.
22. FOLEY, K. M. (1979) Pain syndromes in patients with cancer. In: *Advances in Pain Research*, vol. 2. J. J. Bonica & V. Ventafridda, eds. Raven Press, New York.
23. GOLDSCHEIDER, A. (1894) *Uber den Schmerz*. Hirschwald, Berlin.
24. GREENWALD, H. P. (1991) Interethnic differences in pain perception. *Pain*, 44: 1–7.
25. HAGBARTH, K. E., & KERR, D. I. B. (1954) Central influences on spinal afferent conduction. *J. Neurophysiol.*, 17: 295–307.
26. HILGARD, E. R., & HILGARD, J. R. (1975) *Hypnosis in the Relief of Pain*. Kaufman, Los Altos, CA.
27. JENSEN, T. S., *et al.* (1985) Immediate and long term phantom limb pain in amputees. *Pain*, 21: 267–278.
28. KEELE, K. D. (1957) *Anatomies of Pain*. Blackwell, Oxford.
29. KITZINGER, S. (1984) Episiotomy pain. In: *The Textbook of Pain*, P. D. Wall & R. Melzack, eds. Churchill Livingstone, Edinburgh.
30. KRONER, K., *et al.* (1989) Immediate and long term phantom breast syndrome after mastectomy. *Pain*, 36: 327–334.
31. LINTON, S. J., *et al.* (1989) The secondary prevention of low back pain. *Pain*, 36: 197–208.
32. LIVINGSTON, W. K. (1943) *Pain Mechanisms*. Macmillan, New York.
33. LOESER, J. D. (1980) Low back pain. In: *Pain*, J. J. Bonica, ed. Raven Press, New York.
34. MARCER, D., & DEIGHTON, S. (1988) Intractable pain: A neglected area of medical education in the UK. *J. Roy. Soc. Med.*, 81: 698–700.
35. MARSHALL, H. R. (1894) *Pain, Pleasure and Aesthetics*. Macmillan, London.
36. McGRATH, P. A. (1990) *Pain in Children. Nature, Assessment and Treatment*. Guildford, New York.
37. McGRATH, P. A., & UNRUH, A. M. (1987) *Pain in Children and Adolescents*. Elsevier, Amsterdam.
38. McMAHON, S. B., & WALL, P. D. (1984) Receptive fields of rat lamina I projection cells move to incorporate a nearby region of injury. *Pain*, 19: 235–247.
39. McQUAY, H. J., CARROLL, D., & MOORE, R. A. (1988) Postoperative orthopaedic pain. *Pain*, 33: 291–295.

40. MELZACK, R. (1975) The McGill Pain Questionnaire. *Pain*, 1: 277–299.
41. MELZACK, R. (1984) The myth of painless childbirth. *Pain*, 19: 331–337.
42. MELZACK, R., & WALL, P. D. (1965) Pain mechanisms: A new theory. *Science*, 150: 971–979.
43. MELZACK, R., WALL, P. D., & TY, T. C. (1982) Acute pain in the emergency clinic. *Pain*, 14: 33–43.
44. MENDELL, L. M. (1966) Physiological properties of unmyelinated fibre projections to the spinal cord. *Exp. Neurol.*, 16: 316–332.
45. MENDELL, L. M., & WALL, P. D. (1965) Responses of single dorsal cord cells to peripheral cutaneous unmyelinated fibres. *Nature*, 206: 97–99.
46. MERSKEY, H. (1979) Pain terms. *Pain*, 6: 249–252.
47. MITCHELL, S. W. (1872) Injuries of nerves and their consequences. Lippincott, Philadelphia.
48. MOUNT, B. M. (1989) Psychological and social aspects of cancer pain. In: *The Textbook of Pain*, 2nd ed. P. D. Wall & R. Melzack, eds. Churchill Livingstone, Edinburgh.
49. MOUNTCASTLE, V. B. (1968) *Medical Physiology*, 12th ed. Mosby, St. Louis.
50. MUNLEY, A. (1983) *The Hospice Alternative*. Basic Books, New York.
51. NEAL, H. (1978) *The Politics of Pain*. McGraw-Hill, New York.
52. NOORDENBOS, W. (1959). *Pain*. Elsevier, Amsterdam.
53. OLESEN, J., & EDVINSSON, L. (1988) *Basic Mechanisms of Headache*. Elsevier, Amsterdam.
54. ORNE, M. T., & DINGES, D. F. (1989) Hypnosis. In: *The Textbook of Pain*, 2nd ed., P. D. Wall & R. Melzack, eds. Churchill Livingstone, Edinburgh.
55. SAUNDERS, C. (1989) Pain and impending death. In: *The Textbook of Pain*, 2nd ed. P. D. Wall & R. Melzack, eds. Churchill Livingstone, Edinburgh.
56. SHERMAN, R. A., & SHERMAN C. J. (1985) A comparison of phantom sensations among amputees. *Pain*, 21: 91–97.
57. SHERMAN, R. A., SHERMAN, C. J., & PARKER, L. (1984) Chronic phantom and stump pain among American veterans: Results of a survey. *Pain*, 18: 83–95.
58. SHERRINGTON, C. S. (1906) Integrative action of the nervous system. Scribner, New York.
59. STERNBACH, R. A. (1963) Congenital insensitivity to pain. *Psychol. Bull.*, 60: 252–264.
60. STERNBACH, R. A. (1968) Pain: A psychophysiological analysis. Academic Press, New York.
61. STERNBACH, R. A. (1986a) Survey of pain in the United States. The Nuprin Pain Report. *Clin. J. Pain.*, 2: 49–53.
62. STERNBACH, R. A. (1986b) Pain and "hassles" in the United States. Findings of the Nuprin Pain Report. *Pain*, 27: 69–80.
63. STERNBACH, R. A., & TURSKY, B. (1965) Ethnic differences among housewives in psychophysical and skin potential responses to electric shock. *Psychophysiology*, 1: 241–246.

64. TAUB, A. (1964) Local, segmental and supraspinal interaction with a dorsolateral spinal cutaneous afferent system. *Expl. Neurol.*, 10: 357–374.
65. TAYLOR, H., & CURRAN, N. M. (1985) The Nuprin Report, Louis Harris, New York. (Available by writing to Nuprin Pain Report, P.O. Box 14093, Baltimore, MD 21203.)
66. TWYCROSS, R. G., & LACK, S. A. (1990) *Therapeutics in Terminal Cancer*, 2nd ed. Edward Arnold, London.
67. VALLBO, A. B., & HAGBARTH, K. E. (1968) Activity from skin mechanoreceptors recorded percutaneously in awake human subjects. *Expl. Neurol.*, 21: 270–289.
68. VOUDOURIS, N. J., PECK, C. L., & COLEMAN, G. (1990) The role of conditioning and verbal expectancy in the placebo response. *Pain*, 43: 121–128.
69. WALL, P. D. (1960) Cord cells responding to touch damage and temperature of skin. *J. Neurophysiol.*, 23: 197–210.
70. WALL, P. D. (1967) The laminar organization of dorsal horn and effects of descending impulses. *J. Physiol.*, 188: 403–423.
71. WALL, P. D. (1979) On the relation of injury to pain. *Pain*, 6:253–264.
72. WALL, P. D., & McMAHON, S. B. (1985) Microneuronography and its relation to perceived sensation. *Pain*, 21: 209–229.
73. WALL, P. D., & SWEET, W. H. (1967) Temporary abolition of pain in man. *Science*, 155: 108–109.
74. WORLD HEALTH ORGANIZATION (1990) Cancer pain relief and palliative care. *Technical Report Series* 804: WHO, Geneva.
75. YAKSH, T. L. (1986) *Spinal Afferent Processing*. Plenum Press, New York.
76. ZBOROWSKI, M. (1969) *People in Pain*. Jossey-Bass, San Francisco.
77. ZORZA, R., & ZORZA, V. (1980) *A Way to Die*. Deutsch, London.

Further Reading

Details of the issues discussed in this book can be found in the following four books:

1. For undergraduates in the life sciences and for medical students.
   The Challenge of Pain, revised ed. Ronald Melzack & Patrick D. Wall. Penguin, London, 1988.
2. For MDs and those with professional training.
   Pain, Howard L. Fields. McGraw-Hill, New York, 1987.
3. For detailed discussion of scientific and clinical issues.
   The Textbook of Pain, 2nd ed. Patrick D. Wall & Ronald Melzack, eds. Churchill Livingstone, Edinburgh, 1989.
4. An updated, expanded version of Bonica's classical 1953 book.
   The Management of Pain, 2nd ed. John J. Bonica. Lea & Febiger, Philadelphia, 1990.

Index

Acetylsalicylic acid, 172
Acupuncture, described, 205–209
Addiction, opiates, 183–185
Age level
  migraine and, 10
  osteoarthritis and, 54
  pain and, 12–13
Alacoque, Saint Marguerite Marie, 150
Alcohol, pain behavior and, 159
Alcoholism, peripheral nerve damage pain, 59
Alexandrian school, pain causes, 32
Amputation, 255–256
  depression and, 223
  pain and, 14
  peripheral nerve damage pain, 60
  phantom limb pain, 99–104
Analgesics
  narcotic (opiates), 181–188
  nonsteroidal anti-inflammatory drugs (NSAIDs), 172–175
Anesthesia
  childbirth pain, 88–90
  local, described, 176–179
Antidepressants, described, 180
Antiepileptic drugs, described, 188–189

Antisympathetic therapy, described, 179–180
Anxiety
  pain behavior, 157–159
  psychotherapy, 221
Aristotle, 31, 109–110
Arthritis, back pain, 66
Aspirin, naming of, 172
Attitudes, toward pain, 3–5, 10–11, 263–265
Augustine of Hippo, Saint, 254
Authority, 254–255

Back pain
  pain behavior and, 162
  pain causes, 64–68
  paradoxes in, 105–106
  pregnancy and, 71
Bacterial infection, peripheral nerve damage pain, 59
Balzac, Honoré de, 205
Bard, Philip, 264
Bayer Company, 172, 182
Beecher, Henry K., 94, 97, 101–102, 128
Behavior: see Pain behavior
Behavior therapy, described, 227–228

277

Belief-and-attitude therapies, 215–
        233
    behavior therapy, 227–228
    cognitive therapy, 228
    hypnosis, 229–233
    meditation, 229
    overview of, 215–216
    placebo therapy, 216–220
    psychotherapy, 221–226
    relaxation training, 228–229
Bell, Charles, 118
Berkeley, George, 112
Bone pain, cancer and, 57
Bonica, J. J., 83–84, 128, 144, 236
Bouckoms, A. J., 195–196
Brain
    future research on, 259–260
    mapping of, 115–116
    opiates and, 185–186
    pain center concept, 123
    pain mechanisms and, 115–118
    psychosurgery, 195–196
    senses and, 118–122
Brain tumor, pain signals and, 146–
        147
Bristol Myers Company, 258
Burn pain, pain causes, 47–48
Byron, George Gordon, Lord, 181

Caesar, Julius, 75
Cancer and cancer pain, 18
    advances in treatment of, 13
    hospice programs and, 245–251
    opiates and, 185
    pain causes, 55–58
    pain signals and, 146–147
    radiotherapy/chemotherapy for,
        200–201
    treatment for, 171
    World Health Organization and,
        235–236
Carpal tunnel syndrome, peripheral
        nerve surgery for, 196

Cause and effect relationship,
        medical treatment, 168–171
Cesarean section, childbirth pain
        and, 75–78
Charcot, Jean-Martin, 119–120
Chemotherapy, described, 200–201
Childbirth pain, 69–90
    birth preparation, 71–72
    causes of, 74–75
    historical perspective on, 69–70
    intrusions and, 75–78
    labor pain, 72–74
        first stage, 72–73
        second stage, 73–74
        third stage, 74
    natural childbirth, 85–87
    pregnancy pain, 70–71
    relief of, 87–90
    at risk populations for pain, 82–
        85
    women's comments on, 78–82
Children, pain and, 10
Chiropractics, described, 199–200
Chomsky, Noam, 128
Christianity, moral value myth, 148–
        152
Chronic pain, pain behavior, 155–
        157
Clive, Robert, 181
Cocaine
    addiction to, 183
    medical uses of, 177
Codeine, 182
Cognitive therapy, described, 228
Cold therapy (physiotherapy),
        described, 209–210
Coleridge, Samuel Taylor, 181
Color, senses and, 110
Congenital analgesia, described,
        95–96
Conversion disorder, described,
        225–226
Cordotomy, described, 194–195

Crick, Francis, 126
Crimean War, 91–92
Culture
    acupuncture, 205–209
    childbirth pain and, 73, 76, 83–85
    cross-cultural perspective, 10
    hypnosis and, 231–232
    massage therapy, 210–211
    moral value myth, 148–152
    opium and, 181
    stoicism and, 147–148
Darwin, Charles, 120, 181
Defiance pattern, pain behavior,
        162–163
Democritus, 109
Demography, pain and, 12–13
Depression
    antidepressants for, 180
    pain behavior and, 157–159
    pain clinics and, 239
    psychotherapy for, 221, 222
De Quincey, Thomas, 181
Descartes, René, 32–34, 39, 112–113,
        123, 124, 125
Diabetes, peripheral nerve damage
        pain, 59
Dickens, Charles, 181
Dinesen, Izak, 59
Disc surgery, described, 197–199
DNA, 126
Doctor–patient relationship; see also
        Medical treatment
    crisis in, 263–265
    defiance pattern of pain behavior
        and, 162
    malpractice suits, 162
    medical treatment and, 167–189
    pain clinics and, 237
    responsibility and, 255–256
    sensitivity of, 142–145
Do-it-yourself stimulation therapy,
        described, 203–204
Donne, John, 142

Dorsal column stimulation,
        described, 202–203
Dorsal horn surgery, 194
Dostoyevsky, Feodor, 116
Dreser, Heinrich, 172
Drug addiction, opiates, 183–185
Drug nomenclature, described, 172–
        173
Drugs, pain behavior and, 158–159;
        see also Medical treatment

Eccles, John, 125–126
Economic factors, pain, 11–12
Eisenhower, Dwight D., 49
Elderly
    osteoarthritis, 54
    pain and, 12–13
Eliot, T. S., 209
Epidemiology
    of back pain, 105–106
    of pain, generally, 7–15
Epilepsy, 116
    antiepileptic drugs, 188–189
Episiotomy, childbirth pain and, 78
Esdaile, James, 230
Euripides, 69–70
Exercise therapy, described, 212–214

Ferrier, David, 263
Finneson, Bernard, 218
Folk medicine
    described, 204–205
    movement toward, 253
Franklin, Benjamin, 170
Freud, Sigmund, 88, 177

Galen, 183
Gall, Franz Josef, 116–118
Galvani, Luigi, 119
Gate control
    opiates and, 186
    pain mechanisms, 130–134
Generic drug names, 172–173

Goethe, Johann Wolfgang von, 110
Goldscheider, Albert, 127
Golgi, Camillo, 34–36
Guilt, pain behavior, 157–159, 256

Hahnemann, Samuel, 19
Head, Henry, 263
Headache pain
  pain causes, 62–64
  paradoxes in, 104–105
Heart attack pain, pain causes, 48–52
Heat therapy (physiotherapy),
  described, 209–210
Heberden, William, 48
Heine, Heinrich, 106
Helmholtz, Hermann Ludwig
  Ferdinand von, 110
Holistic medicine, 215; see also
  Belief-and-attitude therapies
Homeopathy, 19
Hospice programs, described, 245–
  251
Hume, David, 112
Huxley, Aldous, 229
Hypnosis, described, 229–233
Hypochondria, described, 224–225
Hysteria: see Conversion disorder

Iatrogenic pain, described, 15
Idiopathic pain, described, 226
Implanted electrode nerve
  stimulation, described, 202
Impulse-triggered prolonged pain
  mechanisms, pain
  mechanisms, 134–135
Induction of labor, childbirth pain
  and, 77–78
Infection, peripheral nerve damage
  pain, 59
Injury: see Traumatic injury
Insurance companies, hospice
  programs and, 251

International Association for the
  Study of Pain, 16

Jackson, Hughlings, 121
John Paul II (Pope), 150
Joint and muscle movement therapy,
  described, 211–212
Justins, Douglas, 237

Kant, Immanuel, 112
Keats, John, 181
Koller, Carl, 88, 177

Labor pain: see Childbirth pain
Laennec, René Théophile, 76
Language
  pain and, 22–25
  pain behavior and, 154–155
La Rochefoucauld, François de, 152
Law, opiates, 183
Leriche, René, 146
Lessing, Doris, 80–81
Lettvin, Jerome, 128
Lewis, C. S., 151, 152, 254
Lewis, Thomas, 263
Liver disease, referred pain, 51
Livingstone, David, 93–94, 97–98
Livingstone, William, 128
Local anesthetics, described, 176–
  179
Low forceps intervention, childbirth
  pain and, 78
Lung cancer, pain signals and, 146

MacDougall, William, 231
Magendie, François, 118
Malaria, 17–18
Malpractice suits, pain behavior
  and, 162
Mangold, Dorothy, 141–142
Marshall, H. R., 144
Massage therapy, described, 210–211

McCulloch, Warren, 128
McGill Pain Questionnaire
    childbirth pain and, 79, 87
    origin of, 22–23
Medical treatment, 167–189
    anesthetics, local, 176–179
    antidepressants, 180
    antiepileptic drugs, 188–189
    antisympathetic therapy, 179–180
    cause and effect relationship, 168–
        171
    drug nomenclature, 172–173
    nonsteroidal anti-inflammatory
        drugs (NSAIDs), 172–175
    opiates (narcotic analgesics), 181–
        188
    overview of, 167–168
    side effects in, 171–172
    steroids, 176
Meditation, described, 229
Melzack, Ronald, 22–23, 86–87,
        127–128, 128, 129
Men, childbirth pain and, 82
Merskey, Harold, 28
Mesmer, Friedrich, 229
Migraine headache
    cross-cultural perspective on, 10
    pain causes, 62–64
    paradoxes in, 104–105
Mind/body relationship
    pain paradoxes, 107
    science and, 116
Mitchell, Weir, 22, 99–100, 105
Montaigne, Michel de, 94
Moral value myth, pain neglect,
        148–152
Morgan, John, 147
Morphine
    brain actions of, 186
    described, 182
Mott, Frederick, 263
Mountcastle, Vernon, 28

Muller, Johannes Petrus, 118–119
Muscle and joint movement therapy,
        described, 211–212
Myocardial infarction: see Heart
        attack

Napoleon (emp. of France), 106, 117–
        118
Narcotic analgesics (opiates),
        described, 181–188
Nasser, Gamal Abdel, 59
National Health Service (NHS), 141–
        142
National Institutes of Health (NIH),
        257
National Science Foundation, 257
Natural childbirth, childbirth pain,
        85–87
Neal, Helen, 16
Needs, sensation and, 111
Nerve fibers
    antisympathetic therapy, 179–180
    pain pathways and, 123
Nerve surgery, described, 192–195
Nervous system anatomy
    historical perspective, 34–39
    single sensory nerve fibers, 38–39
    spinal cord, 39–40
Neurology, 18, 115–116
Neurosis
    conversion disorder, 225–226
    hypochondria, 224–225
Newton, Isaac, 110
Nightingale, Florence, 181
Nixon, Richard M., 205
Nociceptor
    pain definitions and, 29
    pain pathways and, 123
Nonsteroidal anti-inflammatory
        drugs (NSAIDs), described,
        172–175
Noordenbos, William, 128

NSAIDs: *see* Nonsteroidal anti-
    inflammatory drugs
    (NSAIDs)

Opiates (narcotic analgesics),
    described, 181–188
Orthopedic surgery, described, 198–
    199
Orwell, George, 26, 181
Osler, William, 51
Osteoarthritis pain, pain causes,
    52–54
Osteopathy, described, 199–200

Pain
    advances in treatment of, 1–2
    amputation, 14
    attitudes toward, 3–5, 10–11, 18–
        19
    cancer and, 13
    childbirth, 69–90; *see also*
        Childbirth pain
    congenital analgesia, 95–96
    cross-cultural perspective on, 10
    definitions of, 21–29
        experiential, 21–22
        language and, 22–25
        perception and, 27–28
        physical/mental dichotomy, 25–
            26
    economic costs of, 11–12
    epidemiology of, 7–15
    historical perspective on, 17–19
    iatrogenic pain, 15
    painless traumatic injury, 91–95;
        see also Painless traumatic
        injury
    patient-doctor relationship and,
        142–145
    pregnancy pain, 70–71
    public attention and, 15–21
    research in, 2–3, 16–17, 259–261

Pain (*cont.*)
    sources of, 8
    stress and, 8–9
    usefulness of, 145–147, 254
Pain behavior, 153–165
    chronic pain, 155–157
    defiance pattern, 162–163
    described, 153–155
    guilt, anxiety, and depression,
        157–159
    resignation pattern, 164–165
    self-pity pattern, 159–161
Pain causes, 31–68
    Alexandrian school, 32
    back pain, 64–68
    burns, 47–48
    cancer, 55–58
    Cartesian explanations, 32–34
    headache, 62–64
    heart attack, 48–52
    initial causes, 31–32
    nervous system anatomy
        historical perspective, 34–39
        single sensory nerve fibers, 38–
            39
        spinal cord, 39–40
    osteoarthritis, 52–54
    peripheral nerve damage, 58–62
    postoperative pain, 45–47
    rheumatoid arthritis, 54–55
    scratch, 40–42
    toothache, 43–44
    traumatic injury, 44–45
    twisted ankle, 42–43
Pain center, concept development,
    122–123
Pain clinics, 236–244
    case histories, 237–244
    multidisciplinary focus of, 236– 237
Pain (journal), 16
Painless traumatic injury
    congenital analgesia, 95–96

Painless traumatic injury (*cont.*)
  examples of, 91–95
  explanations for, 97–99
Pain mechanisms, 109–140
  external and internal realities,
    110–112
  gate control, 130–134
  hypotheses of, 115–126
  impulse-triggered prolonged pain
    mechanisms, 134–135
  instantaneous reality, 112–113
  primary sensations, 109–110
  recent discoveries in
    described, 126–130
    impact of, 137–140
  sensation/perception order, 113–
    114
  sensation prolonged, 114–115
  transport-controlled prolonged
    pain mechanisms, 134–135
Pain neglect, 20, 141–152
  doctor–patient relationship, 142–
    145
  moral value myth, 148–152
  pain utility and, 145–146
  stoicism and, 147–148
Pain pathway, concept development,
  122–123
Paracelsus, 229
Paraplegia, 19
Paré, Ambroise, 100
Pasteur, Louis, 17
Patient-controlled analgesia (PCA),
  187
Patient–doctor relationship: *see*
  Doctor–patient relationship
Pavlov, I. P., 39, 219
Perception
  pain definitions and, 27–28
  sensation precedes, 113–114
Peripheral nerve damage pain, pain
  causes, 58–62

Personality, pain behavior, chronic
  pain, 155–157
Phantom limb pain, described, 99–
  104
Physical/mental dichotomy, pain
  definitions, 25–26
Physicians: *see* Doctor–patient
  relationship
Physiotherapy, described, 209–210
Pitts, Walter, 128
Placebo effect
  belief-and-attitude therapies, 215
  historical perspective on, 168
  research in, 168–169
Placebo reactors, 125
Placebo therapy, described, 216–
  220
Popper, Karl, 125–126
Postoperative pain
  opiates and, 185–187
  pain causes, 45–47
Posture, pregnancy and, 71
Pregnancy pain, described, 70–71
Pressure relief surgery, described,
  196–199
Proprionic acids, 173
Psychiatry; *see also* Pain behavior
  defiance pattern of pain behavior
    and, 163
  development of, 115–116
Psychogenic pain disorder,
  described, 226
Psychosurgery, described, 195–196
Psychotherapy, described, 221–226

Radiotherapy, described, 200–201
Ramon y Cajal, Santiago, 34–36, 39,
  115
Read, Grantly Dick, 85–86
Reagan, Ronald, 92–93
Referred pain, heart attack pain, 50–
  51

Relaxation training, described, 228–229

Religion, moral value myth, 148–152

Resignation pattern, pain behavior, 164–165

Responsibility, doctor–patient relationship and, 255–256

Rheumatoid arthritis pain, causes, 54–55

Riley–Day syndrome, 257

Roosevelt, Eleanor, 84

Saunders, Cicely, 105, 246, 250

Scratch pain, pain causes, 40–42

Self-pity pattern, pain behavior, 159–161

Sensation
instantaneous reality, 112–113
perception follows, 113–114
prolonged sensation, 114–115
senses contrasted, 111

Senses
brain and, 118–122
external and internal realities, 110–112
pain mechanisms and, 109–110
sensation contrasted, 111
subdivision of, 122–124

Sex differences, migraine and, 10

Shakespeare, William, 24

Shannon, Claude, 128

Shelley, Percy Bysshe, 24, 181

Sherrington, Charles, 39

Shingles, peripheral nerve damage pain, 59

Silent heart attack, pain and, 51–52

Simpson, James Young, 88

Skin senses, research in, 110

Slipped disc, back pain, 64–66, 106

Spencer, Herbert, 121

Spiller, W. H., 123

Spinal cord
damage to, 19
disc surgery, 197–199
opiates and, 186
osteopathy/chiropractics, 199–200
pain mechanisms and, 118
pain pathways and, 123

Spinal stenosis, back pain, 66

Staining methods, brain anatomy and, 119

Sternbach, Richard, 8–9, 157, 231

Steroids, described, 176

Stimulation therapy, 201–214
acupuncture, 205–209
do-it-yourself stimulation, 203–204
dorsal column stimulation, 202–203
exercise, 212–214
folk medicine, 204–205
implanted electrode nerve stimulation, 202
joint and muscle movement, 211–212
massage, 210–211
overview of, 201–202
physiotherapy, 209–210
transcutaneous electrical nerve stimulation (TENS), 202
vibration, 203

Stoicism, pain neglect and, 147–148

Stone, Edmund, 17, 172

Stress
pain and, 8–9
psychotherapy, 221–222

Surgery: see Postoperative pain

Surgical treatment, 192–199
nerve surgery, 192–195
pressure relief, 196–199
psychosurgery, 195–196

Suso, Henry, 149

Sweet, William, 201

Sydenham, Thomas, 181, 183
Symptomatic medicine, 18
Syphilis, peripheral nerve damage
     pain, 59

Tension, psychotherapy, 221
Tension headache
   pain causes, 62–64
   paradoxes in, 104–105
Terminal illness, hospice programs,
     245–251
Thebaine, 182
Therapeutic community, need for,
     265–268
Therapy: see Belief-and-attitude
     therapies; Chemotherapy;
     Chiropractics; Medical
     treatment; Osteopathy;
     Radiotherapy; Stimulation
     therapy; Surgical treatment;
     Therapeutic community
Tolerance, opiates, 184, 187
Tolstoy, Leo, 91–92, 100
Toothache pain, causes, 43–44
Torture, 26–27
Transcutaneous electrical nerve
     stimulation (TENS)
   described, 202
   do-it-yourself therapy, 203–204
Transport-controlled prolonged pain
     mechanisms, pain
     mechanisms, 134–135
Traumatic injury
   pain and, 13
   pain causes, 44–45
   painless, 91–95; see also Painless
     traumatic injury
   pain utility and, 145–146
   peripheral nerve damage pain, 60

Traumatic injury (cont.)
   scratch, 40–42
Treatment: see Belief-and-attitude
     therapies; Chemotherapy;
     Chiropractics; Medical
     treatment; Osteopathy;
     Radiotherapy; Stimulation
     therapy; Surgical treatment;
     Therapeutic community
Trigeminal nerve surgery, 193
Twisted ankle pain, causes, 42–43

Vibration therapy, described, 203
Victoria (queen of England), 87–88
Viral infection, peripheral nerve
     damage pain, 59
Virchow, Rudolf, 17
Volta, Count Alessandro, 119
von Frey, Max, 122, 127

Wall, Patrick D., 128
Warfare, 13–14
   painless injury and, 91–92, 94
   phantom limb pain, 101–102
Watson, James, 126
Whittington Pain Program, 240–244
Wilder, Thornton, 160
Women, childbirth pain comments
     of, 78–82
Wordsworth, William, 24
World Health Organization
   cancer pain and, 235–236
   opiates and, 183
Wynn-Parry, C. E., 196

Zola, Emile, 92, 98
Zorza, Rosemary, 248
Zorza, Victor, 248